"We wish this book had been there to share w
we have taught who wondered about the brair
panion for both students interested in psychol
exciting specialty, clinical neuropsychology, and all of us that want to provide
direction and wisdom about the wonders of the brain and the many opportunities for careers that accompany a vocation dedicated to the brain and those
afflicted with brain disease."

Antonio E. Puente, *Ph.D., ABN, AAPdN, Past-president,*
American Psychological Association, Professor of Psychology,
University of North Carolina Wilmington
and
Antonio N. Puente, *Ph.D., ABPP-CN, Assistant Professor of*
Psychiatry and Neurology, George Washington University

"Drs. Schaefer and Bertisch have filled a void in American education by
targeting an intriguing STEM career in clinical neuropsychology as an as-
pirational goal for high school and for undergraduate college students. The
authors have performed a masterful job in providing a detailed and systematic
pathway to eventual success in this pursuit at a stage in student's educational
development often devoid of specific guidance. This book not only will be
invaluable to students and to their families, it will have the extended benefit
of opening a pipeline for qualified professionals to treat the many health and
behavioral problems confronting our society across the lifespan from childhood through advanced age."

Allan Yozawitz, *Ph.D., ABPP-CN, Board Certified in Clinical*
Neuropsychology, Fellow, American Psychological Association

"Schaefer & Bertisch have created an accessible and illuminating guide!
Working with the Brain in Psychology: Considering Careers in Neuropsychol-
ogy is engaging, clear, and covers an extensive range of topics. This is an essential book for any student considering career paths in clinical fields. It is an
especially valuable resource for faculty and academic advisors to share with
their students. The optimism, candor, and balanced perspective in this guide
will allow readers to return to this book often as they develop their careers."

Barbara J. Luka, *Ph.D., Psychology & Integrative Neuroscience*
Academic Advisor, Binghamton University

Working with the Brain in Psychology

Working with the Brain in Psychology: Considering Careers in Neuropsychology seeks to assist students in their career exploration, by introducing them early, in the contemplative stage of career planning, to the fascinating specialty of psychology known as neuropsychology. The text spends considerable time differentiating neuropsychology from alternative career paths, and provides personal accounts, contributions from neuropsychologists in various settings, and case examples of different patient populations to illustrate what it is like to train to become and work as a neuropsychologist.

This text begins by describing what neuropsychology is, how it is situated within psychology, and for whom it could be a good fit. Suggestions are provided about how to engage in self-assessment in order to help choose a career. It goes on to review over a dozen similar and overlapping careers to illustrate how neuropsychology stands out. Quotes by professional neuropsychologists bring to life what "a day in the life" looks like in different settings, and the kinds of populations with whom neuropsychologists work are illustrated with case examples. This book then outlines how one becomes a neuropsychologist, including how to re-specialize from a different field. It also gives an honest appraisal of potential challenges that come with this career and ends with anticipated future directions in the profession to look forward to.

This book will be useful primarily for psychology-minded undergraduates and college graduates thinking of going on to graduate school for psychology, as well as for high school students interested in the brain and psychology. This book is further aimed at those considering a change of career from a related field into neuropsychology, as well as the guidance counselors and college career centers that assist with career planning.

Lynn A. Schaefer, Ph.D., ABPP-CN, is Director of Neuropsychology at Nassau University Medical Center. She is a fellow of the APA and National Academy of Neuropsychology, and co-Chair of the Scholastic Committee for the New York State Association of Neuropsychology. Her interests include remediation of neurobehavioral disorders, educational outreach, and capacity.

Hilary C. Bertisch, Ph.D., ABPP-CN, is Assistant Professor of Psychiatry at the Donald and Barbara Zucker School of Medicine at Hofstra/Northwell. She is a Fellow of the National Academy of Neuropsychology and co-Chair of the Scholastic Committee of the New York State Association of Neuropsychology. Her interests are in the areas of psychosis and brain injury.

Working with the Brain in Psychology

Considering Careers
in Neuropsychology

**Lynn A. Schaefer and
Hilary C. Bertisch**

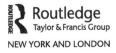

Routledge
Taylor & Francis Group

NEW YORK AND LONDON

Designed cover image: © Getty Images

First published 2024
by Routledge
605 Third Avenue, New York, NY 10158

and by Routledge
4 Park Square, Milton Park, Abingdon, Oxon, OX14 4RN

Routledge is an imprint of the Taylor & Francis Group, an informa business

Library of Congress Cataloging-in-Publication Data
Names: Schaefer, Lynn A., author. | Bertisch, Hilary C., author.
Title: Working with the brain in psychology : considering careers in
neuropsychology / Lynn A. Schaefer, Hilary C. Bertisch.
Description: New York, NY : Routledge, 2024. | Includes bibliographical
references and index. |
Identifiers: LCCN 2023027680 (print) | LCCN 2023027681 (ebook) |
ISBN 9781032325361 (hardback) | ISBN 9781032325378 (paperback) |
ISBN 9781003315513 (ebook)
Subjects: LCSH: Neuropsychology—Vocational guidance.
Classification: LCC QP360 .S325 2024 (print) | LCC QP360 (ebook) |
DDC 612.8023—dc23/eng/20230712
LC record available at https://lccn.loc.gov/2023027680
LC ebook record available at https://lccn.loc.gov/2023027681

ISBN: 9781032325361 (hbk)
ISBN: 9781032325378 (pbk)
ISBN: 9781003315513 (ebk)

DOI: 10.4324/9781003315513

Typeset in Times New Roman
by codeMantra

Access the Support Material: www.routledge.com/9781032325361

To my husband Marc, for love and support over 30 years, and for being my biggest cheerleader.

To our twins. My first book (my dissertation) was dedicated to our children, William and Elizabeth.

My second book was dedicated to Elizabeth and William.

This book is dedicated to William and Elizabeth, Elizabeth and William. There, you're even! Love, Mom

–LAS

To Izzy and Remi for their love and support of my work on a daily basis, and to my parents and sister without whom I could not have gotten this far.

To Sydney and Taylor who are the future of the field, and to Ryder in the work that he chooses one day.

–HB

In Memoriam

Dr. Peter J. Donovick

Professor Emeritus, Binghamton University

For introducing us to the field of Neuropsychology

Contents

Contributors

Valerie Abel, Psy.D., ABPP, VA New York Harbor Healthcare System, Brooklyn campus, Brooklyn, NY

Bridget Amatore, Ph.D., John Jay College of Criminal Justice, City University of New York, New York, NY, and Teachers College, Columbia University, New York, NY

Beth C. Arredondo, Ph.D., ABPP-CN, Ochsner Health Center, Covington, LA

Hilary C. Bertisch, Ph.D., ABPP-CN, Northwell Health, Zucker Hillside Hospital, Glen Oaks, NY, and the Donald and Barbara Zucker School of Medicine at Hofstra/Northwell, Hempstead, NY

Sid Binks, Ph.D., ABPP-CN, Sid Binks & Associates: Forensic Neuropsychological Services, Washington, DC

Cindy L. Breitman, Ph.D., ABPP-CN, Behavioral and Neuropsychological Consultants, LLP, New York, NY and Rockville Centre, NY

Alison Cernich, Ph.D., ABPP-CN, Eunice Kennedy Shriver National Institute of Child Health and Human Development, National Institute of Health, Bethesda, MD

Susan D. Croll, Ph.D., Neuroscience, Regeneron Pharmaceuticals, Tarrytown, NY

Kristen Dams-O'Connor, Ph.D., Brain Injury Research Center, Department of Rehabilitation Medicine and Department of Neurology, Icahn School of Medicine at Mount Sinai, NY

Claire Kalpakjian, Ph.D., MS, FACRM, Department of Physical Medicine and Rehabilitation Medicine, Michigan Medicine, University of Michigan, Ann Arbor, MI

Kristine T. Kingsley, Psy.D., ABPP, Institute of Cognitive and Emotional Wellness, New Rochelle, NY

Linda S. LaMarca, Ph.D., ABPP-CN, Glen Cove, NY, and Derner School of Psychology, Adelphi University, Garden City, NY

Gianna Locascio, Psy.D., ABPP, Department of Neurology, NYU Langone Health, Brooklyn, NY

Luba Nakhutina, Ph.D., ABPP-CN, Department of Neurology, SUNY Downstate Health Sciences University, Brooklyn, NY and Comprehensive Neuropsychology Services, P.C., New York, NY

Lawrence Pick, Ph.D., ABPP-CN, Department of Psychology, Gallaudet University, Washington, DC

Joseph Rath, PhD., Department of Psychology, Rusk Rehabilitation, NYU Langone Medical Center, New York, NY

Alice Saperstein, Ph.D., Department of Psychiatry, Columbia University Irving Medical Center, New York, NY, and New York State Office of Mental Health

Lynn A. Schaefer, Ph.D., ABPP-CN, Nassau University Medical Center, East Meadow, NY

David Tulsky, Ph.D., Center for Health Assessment Research and Translation, University of Delaware, Newark, DE

Chriscelyn M. Tussey, Psy.D., ABPP, Metropolitan Forensic & Neuropsychological Consultation, PLLC, New York, NY, and New York University Grossman School of Medicine, New York, NY

Preface and Acknowledgements

Dr. Schaefer and Dr. Bertisch met in 2007, when they both worked in the outpatient Neurorehabilitation Service at Rusk Rehabilitation of New York University Langone Medical Center. As it turns out, both graduated with their undergraduate degrees (several years apart) from Binghamton University, a public research university center in upstate New York. One topical point of interest is that the campus of Binghamton University is actually shaped like a brain and the main road is referred to as "The Brain." It is here that each began their career path toward neuropsychology.

Over the years, Dr. Schaefer would mentor and give talks to undergraduate students about neuropsychology as a potential career. In 2018, she and Dr. Bertisch formed the Scholastic Committee of the New York State Association of Neuropsychology (NYSAN), of which Drs. Schaefer and Bertisch are Co-Chairs. The mission of NYSAN's Scholastic Committee is to educate students of all ages about the specialty of neuropsychology. Toward that end, the Scholastic Committee, at times in conjunction with the New York Neuropsychology Group (NYNG), would host educational outreach events to undergraduate students (and occasionally high school students) about what it is like to work as a neuropsychologist and how to get into the specialty. These outreach events included panel discussions, Q&A sessions, and individual presentations. This book is, in part, an outgrowth of the work of the Scholastic Committee. The aims are many: 1) to consolidate and put into writing the themes and substance of our talks, 2) to reach a larger audience, including students outside of New York State (and perhaps the U.S.), 3) to explain how we came to the specialty of neuropsychology individually, 4) to include discussion about the *contemplative* stage of choosing neuropsychology as a career (including the self-analysis, decision-making, and comparing of similar careers, etc.), and 5) to act as an "academic advisor" of sorts for how to get into the specialty. Essentially, we tried to write the type of book we wished we had when we were exploring career options and considering graduate school. This book will hopefully also be helpful to those considering a change of career from a related field into neuropsychology.

We thank profusely all of the students who provided us feedback and input regarding their concerns and questions, our professional contributors who gave us some insight into their work, and our families for their encouragement and ongoing support. We promise to take at least a small break before starting any new big projects.

We offer a tremendous thanks to Lucy Kennedy, Senior Publisher at Routledge, for her trust and backing of this project. Thanks also goes to Lakshay Gaba at Taylor & Francis, for superb organization and coordination of the myriad technical aspects of publishing a text.

We thank the volume of mentors, colleagues, and friends who have allowed us to reach a point in our careers where writing such a book has been possible. Lastly, we also acknowledge each other for creating an environment of support, encouragement, and creativity where this book, as well as all of the initiatives of the NYSAN Scholastic Committee, can be a success for future students in the specialty.

It is our hope that this book will introduce you, the student, to the fascinating specialty of neuropsychology, assist you in your career exploration, answer burning questions, and quell some anxiety. We wish you luck and enjoyment in whichever path you choose.

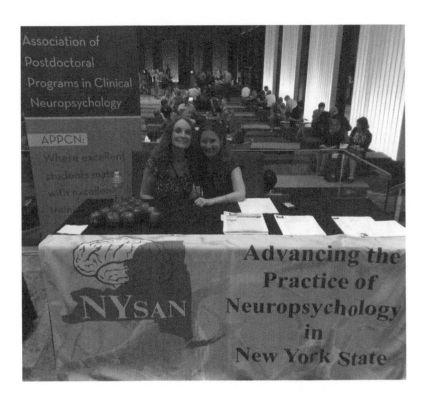

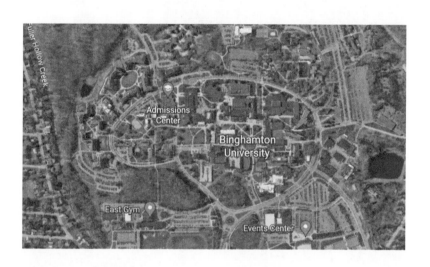

1 What Is Neuropsychology and How Do I Know if It's the Career for Me?

Are you a psychology major who loves the brain? Or a neuroscience major interested in human cognition and consciousness? Perhaps you love both psychology and biology courses, whether in high school or in college, but don't know how to combine the two. Or maybe you are intrigued by the previous topics and think perhaps you would like to see "patients," but are not sure you want to go to medical school. If any of these apply, you've picked up the right book.

This text is for those who are interested in or are considering **neuropsychology** as a career. It may be a specialty that you never heard of until now. Many students have told us that they did not receive much exposure to neuropsychology at the undergraduate level (and certainly not before that). Neuropsychology is a specialty of **psychology** and is "the area of research and clinical practice characterizing the relationship between brain structure/brain function (including clinical disease and syndromes) and behavior" (Loring & Bowden, 2015, p. 259). It is a fascinating and rewarding area of study and practice, although as neuropsychologists we may be a bit biased. Nevertheless, our hope is to introduce students to this specialty as they are exploring and making decisions with regard to career planning.

This book will discuss what neuropsychology is and for whom it is a good fit, review many similar and overlapping careers and how neuropsychology stands out, describe what "a day in the life" of a neuropsychologist looks like in different settings, the kinds of populations with whom neuropsychologists work, and how to become one. We will also discuss some potential challenges with this career, before ending on an optimistic note. This book will not review the history and origin of neuropsychology; this information is available elsewhere (e.g., Bellone & Van Patten, 2021; Bogousslavsky et al., 2019). Instead, we wanted the focus to be on career path selection. Throughout, we have sought to incorporate answers to student questions that have been posed when we have presented this topic to student groups. Ultimately, we remember how difficult it was to choose a career and, given how satisfied and excited we are about our choices, would like to share what we have learned in the hopes of helping current students in their contemplation, exploration, and decision-making.

DOI: 10.4324/9781003315513-1

While you may not have heard much about neuropsychology until now, you probably have been exposed to the discipline of psychology, whether in high school or college. Next, we will briefly introduce the broad field of psychology and its different specialties, and how neuropsychology is situated within psychology. Of note, terms that are in bold are defined in the Glossary included in the back of the book.

How Does Neuropsychology Fit Within Psychology?

Psychology is the study of the mind and behavior, and is a very broad subject. One can go into a number of different careers within psychology. Generally, to become a psychologist, you need to have a graduate degree. However, psychology is an extremely flexible subject and even with an undergraduate degree in psychology, there are a number of opportunities (Kuther & Morgan, 2019; Craig, 2017). Some specialties within psychology are more applied or clinically oriented and prepare you to work with patients or clients, such as clinical psychology, counseling psychology, school psychology, forensic psychology, and industrial-organizational psychology. Others are more research oriented, such as experimental psychology, cognitive psychology, social psychology or developmental psychology. Professional psychologists in both clinical and research specialties can also teach students at the undergraduate and graduate levels.

Neuropsychology is a small specialty of psychology; most psychologists are not neuropsychologists. Neuropsychology is a specialty for students interested in studying the biological and neurological underpinnings of behavior, and the intersection between psychology and biology (i.e., the brain). Coursework in neuropsychology can also sometimes be referred to as psychobiology, biopsychology, **behavioral neuroscience**, or physiological psychology. These terms are typically reserved for courses, and also fields, that focus more on the research aspects of the brain-behavior relationship. Clinical neuropsychology is a specialty of clinical psychology specializing in **neuroscience**. Therefore, it is the applied form of neuropsychology. Some alternative careers in applied psychology will be discussed in Chapter 2.

Clinical neuropsychologists see patients across the lifespan for cognitive assessment, diagnosis, treatment, and/or rehabilitation (see also Chapter 3 for discussion of what a clinical neuropsychologist does). So, you get to work with and help people. In addition to clinical, research, and/or teaching roles, neuropsychologists are also experts in brain health, and can advocate for public health issues, such as concussion prevention, insurance coverage, and care disparities.

There are also a number of subspecialties even within clinical neuropsychology. For example, some neuropsychologists further specialize in a specific age range (**pediatric neuropsychology**; geriatric neuropsychology), focus on expert testimony or work with prison populations (forensic neuropsychology), work primarily with disabled individuals or those with brain injury (rehabilitation neuropsychology), or limit their practice to a specific population or setting (see also Chapters 3 and 4). Some of these subspecialties overlap with other, similar specialties of psychology (see Chapter 2).

Neuropsychology is a good choice if you enjoy studying psychology, find the brain fascinating, and like research (while you will be conducting research at least through graduate school, you will be reading journals to stay abreast of new developments in the subject throughout your career). It is both an intellectually stimulating and rewarding specialty.

How Does One Become Interested in the Specialty?

This is not a one-size-fits-all answer. The path to neuropsychology is different for everyone, although there are likely some commonalities. Most neuropsychologists enter the specialty with an interest in psychology and/or biology. Often people have a hard time deciding between the two, and may struggle with the choice between going to medical school or graduate school to earn a doctoral degree in psychology. Neuropsychology is a perfect blend of these two fields! As we will describe in Chapter 4, some neuropsychologists became interested in this work because they wanted to focus on a certain diagnosis or medical condition, some like a specific age group, and others wanted to work within certain communities where a particular diagnosis or condition is more common. Some may have had volunteer, work, or personal family experience with brain injury, dementia and/or mental illness, and wanted to learn more and be able to help patients with those conditions.

One of the authors (LAS) came to neuropsychology much like the first paragraph of this book described. She loved the subjects of biology and psychology, wanted to better understand the brain, and was attracted to possibly working with patients. As a high school student, she had kept a cow's brain in a jar of formaldehyde on her desk (this was an extra credit assignment for a biology course) and had volunteered at a hospital working with older adults and those with dementia. At the time, her college did not have a neuroscience major, so she started as a biology/pre-med major, also taking classes in psychology, chemistry, and calculus. As mentioned in the Preface, the main road around the campus was shaped like a brain! While she enjoyed and excelled in her biology and psychology courses, she did not find chemistry nearly as stimulating. Meanwhile, as a sophomore, she became involved in two psychology laboratories volunteering as a research assistant and found she really liked and appreciated conducting research. She also served as a teaching assistant (TA) for one of her psychology classes. The deciding factor was taking a course in Physiological Psychology (sometimes called Behavioral Neuroscience). A psychology class, this course focused on the brain and nervous system's role in behavior and cognitive processes, such as sleep, sensation and perception, emotion, **learning** and memory, and communication, as well as psychiatric and neurological disorders. Psychology became the chosen major and career path, and she was even elected to Psi Chi, the Psychology Honor Society. She was especially fortunate to have been exposed to neuropsychology in an elective seminar her junior year. Ultimately, she completed her Ph.D. at the City University of New York (CUNY) Neuropsychology program at Queens College.

Other people come into the specialty by way of their interest in a particular condition or illness that impacts the brain. The other author (HB) found neuropsychology by way of her specific interest in schizophrenia. After she was already in a doctoral program in clinical psychology at Fairleigh Dickinson University, she came to understand that schizophrenia and related diagnoses are conditions of the brain that often cause difficulties with thinking or "**cognition**," in addition to the psychiatric symptoms that define the diagnosis. It therefore made sense to pursue a path to neuropsychology that would allow her to better understand the problems with thinking, what causes this to happen in the brain, and how to help patients with these cognitive difficulties in treatment for their schizophrenia. She later extended this work to people with other brain-related diagnoses. Chapter 4 provides an overview of most brain-related diagnoses that have both clinical and cognitive symptoms and are therefore relevant to a career in neuropsychology.

As you can see, there are different paths to neuropsychology. Some people arrive by way of psychology, and some via neurobiology or neuroscience. Common **academic** interests, however, would include courses not only in psychology, biology and neuroscience, but also cognitive psychology, philosophy, statistics and research methods, and possibly other social sciences such as anthropology or sociology. In fact, since one becomes a neuropsychologist by first achieving a doctorate in psychology, many of the aforementioned subjects are required prerequisites for applying to graduate school (more about this discussed in Chapter 5).

Helping You Choose a Career

But how does one know which profession to go into? Choosing a career can feel exciting, but it can also feel overwhelming, stressful, and anxiety-producing. You may worry about which is the "right" career for you, or fear having regrets that you chose poorly. You may also be getting some pressure from parents, professors, or others about what you are going to do with your life, which only adds to the angst. Since any kind of graduate work is going to be an investment of time and money, the stakes are understandably high. However, we are big believers that, just like there probably isn't only one romantic partner in the whole entire world with whom you are "meant" to be, there are likely a variety of similar careers which would utilize your skills and make you equally happy. Hopefully that eases your mind a bit. Further, career planning can be a process, which sometimes changes over time. So, no need for a quick decision. We will review alternative career choices and describe their similarities and differences to neuropsychology in Chapter 2. Of course, knowledge is power, and the more you know about yourself and your available options, the better. Some people even go on to have multiple different careers during their lifetime. For those looking to transition into neuropsychology from a related field, we will discuss how to do this in Chapter 5.

In order to help choose, we recommend a few steps which can be done in any order including: self-assessment, reading, any practical experiences that you can glean, and speaking to others.

Self-Assessment (aka, Getting to Know Yourself)

In terms of knowing yourself, there are a variety of factors to consider. These include not only your academic interests, but your personality and abilities/skills as well. Just because you love studying a topic doesn't mean that it is necessarily a good fit for you or that you have aptitude in the area. You will want to honestly assess your strengths and weaknesses, as well as your work values, goals, and desired lifestyle. In addition, you will want to reflect on your tolerance for additional years of schooling. You may aspire to earn the title "Doctor," but this requires a huge time investment and is likely alone not a strong enough motivator. For a doctorate, this can be 5–7 years beyond undergraduate work. These are years that it may cost money for tuition, and years that you are still in school while peers are out working and earning money. Speaking of money, you can make a comfortable living as a neuropsychologist (see more in Chapter 5), but you will not become rich; there are certainly occupations that do not require a doctorate where you can make more money, such as in business or finance. Finally, a degree in psychology can be emotionally taxing, especially when dealing with challenging patients and those who have suffered traumas and injuries or illnesses to their brains. Ensure that you have the maturity and are emotionally grounded enough to handle these situations and cases, even if that requires working through issues or problems with your own psychotherapist, and using supervision during your training.

Self-assessment can be formal or informal, or a combination of both. In high school, you can start with your school's guidance counselor. Many colleges and universities also have career centers or advising whereby one can meet with individual counselors or undergo a self-assessment of interests, personality, preferred work environment, etc. Alternatively, private career and job consultants or counselors can also provide assessments for these purposes. Although the **reliability** and **validity** of these types of instruments have been scientifically questioned (Gati & Asulin-Peretz, 2011), they can still provide a student with some approximate information about themselves to use for the purposes of choosing a major or considering a career (or even selecting the type of setting where they would ultimately like to work). For example, while there are many different types of assessments, some of the more commonly used at universities and by career counselors (we asked around) include the

Holland Code, the Myers-Briggs Type Indicator (MBTI), and the Big Five personality traits. A very brief description of each follows, but one can obtain much more information from their school's career or guidance office, or the tests' websites. Of note, websites for many of the below resources are listed in the accompanying eResources for this book.

The Holland Code is based on a theory developed by psychologist Dr. John Holland (1973), whereby one's interests are rated out of six types: Realistic, Investigative, Social, Artistic, Enterprising and Conventional. The first letters of a person's top three types form the code, which can then be used to match compatible occupations. Several job-search sites use the Holland Code, such as O*NET online, developed by the U.S. Department of Labor. Their website is: www.onetonline.org. O*NET is a free online resource for career exploration. Their Interest Profiler uses the Holland Code. In 2022, Dr. Schaefer took part in data collection for O*NET for the specialty of Neuropsychology. Another instrument, the Strong Interest Inventory, also uses the Holland Code. If not available free from their school, one can also obtain their code by taking the test online for a small fee. According to O*NET, the interest code that best matches Neuropsychology is "I-S-A", or Investigative, Social and Artistic. This makes sense, as a neuropsychologist is part detective and part helper; a certain amount of creativity is also required for the job.

The Myers-Briggs Type Indicator (MBTI; Myers et al., 2009) is a tool for self-reflection that has been used by Fortune 100 companies to maximize team effectiveness. It can be taken online for a fee. There are also similar tests, based on this, available for free online. It yields one of 16 "personality types" based on four letter dichotomies, with four corresponding cognitive functions. The letter dichotomies include: Extraverted (E) vs. Introverted (I), Intuitive (N) vs Sensory (S), Feeling (F) vs. Thinking (T), and Perceiving (P) vs. Judging (J). There have been many criticisms of the Myers-Briggs (i.e., Pittenger, 2005; Stromberg & Caswell, 2015; Stein & Swan, 2019), citing that this was developed theoretically and is not scientifically based; its reliability has been questioned. However, other studies have found some associations between particular types and satisfaction in specific occupations (Yang et al., 2016) or more validity in specific populations, such as college students (Randall et al., 2017). In general, according to this theory, psychologists (including neuropsychologists) tend to be higher on the Intuitive (N) type rather than the Sensory (S) type; intuitives are thought to focus more on ideas, possibilities, abstractions, theories, and the big picture, whereas sensory types are more concrete and focus on details. There is also a slight preference for Feeling (F) over Thinking (T). Other than that, there is a mix of the other letter dichotomies, and any personality type can become a psychologist. Those with an Extraverted (E) preference, however, may feel isolated working exclusively in a solo practice, so knowing your type can be helpful for choosing work setting as well. The book *Do What You Are* by Tieger, Barron and Tieger (2014) helps with career choice though the use of these personality types. If nothing else, it is another tool for self-awareness and assessing likes and dislikes, personal strengths, and weaknesses.

The Big 5 personality test is supposed to measure traits such as openness, conscientiousness, extroversion, agreeableness, and neuroticism (Costa & McCrae, 1992; Furnham, 2021). This can be taken through a career counselor or on various websites. The Big 5 has been studied empirically and its reliability and validity has been demonstrated, as opposed to the MBTI (Hurtz & Donovan, 2000). Psychologists in general tend to be high on agreeableness, defined as being empathetic and finding pleasure in helping others and working with people. They would likely also score high on openness and conscientiousness, and low on neuroticism.

On tools like O*NET, you can also search for jobs that best reflect your interests, skills and values. Values in this context include needs and motivations including: Achievement, Independence, Recognition, Relationships, Support, and Working Conditions. According to O*NET, the work values that best match Neuropsychology are Independence, Recognition, and Achievement. Specifically, this is an occupation that allows one to work on their own and make decisions, offers potential for leadership and can be considered prestigious, and allows one to use their strongest abilities, giving them a feeling of accomplishment. Projected growth in the specialty, at least through 2026, was considered "bright" and faster than average, indicating that there is a need for our services and a low rate of unemployment.

A related website, also sponsored by the U.S. Department of Labor, is CareerOneStop https://www.careeronestop.org/, which can help with career exploration, training and job search. This site also contains a self-assessment of interests, skills, and work values.

Again, a few different, but related, careers may check all the boxes for the needs you identify, and that's OK (even better, because then you'll have options). Try to tune in to what you want and need in a career, including goals and lifestyle, but keep an open mind. Ultimately, you will want to do something you're passionate about that is a good fit and also best utilizes your skills and what you do well.

Read All You Can

There are many books and websites available that can help you choose a career. Some are more general and give suggestions for overall career decision-making. Others are for learning more about specific subjects and jobs. Especially if you haven't had a formal class in neuropsychology, you can read more about the specialty with texts such as: *Fundamentals of Human Neuropsychology* by Kolb and Whishaw (2009), *Neuropsychological Assessment* by Lezak et al. (2012), or the *Textbook of Clinical Neuropsychology* by Morgan and Ricker (2017), to name just a few. Check out your library to see if you can borrow any of these.

Also recommended are books about interesting "cases" in the specialty such as *The Man Who Mistook His Wife for a Hat* by Oliver Sacks (or any of his books; Sacks, 1985/2021) or *The Banana Lady* (Kertesz, 2006). Other, more personal accounts of brain-behavior illness or injury include *Over My Head* (Osborn, 2000) or *My Stroke of Insight* (Taylor, 2017), about brain injury and stroke, respectively. The book series *After Brain Injury: Survivor Stories* (link in eResources) contains multiple volumes offering real-life perspectives from survivors of various brain injuries and illnesses, all still living with the consequences. If you are devouring the stories, neuropsychology just may be the specialty for you! Finally, books like the one you're currently reading, such as Bellone & Van Patten's *Becoming a Neuropsychologist: Advice and Guidance for Students and Trainees* (2021) or Block's *The Neuropsychologist's Roadmap: A Training and Career Guide* (2021) can help. Both of these books guide you through the process of becoming a neuropsychologist, assuming you've already decided on a career; this book, in contrast, hopes to help more with the initial exploration, comparison, and decision-making.

Virtually, there are plenty of websites about neuropsychology, too numerous to mention, and there are even YouTube videos that can show you the "day in the life" of many different professions, neuropsychology included.

Get Some Experience

You can try to "shadow," observe, or at least interview, some people in the professions you are interested in to see if you like how they spend their days. Sometimes shadowing or observing is difficult or prohibited, particularly in a hospital setting where there are privacy issues, but it can't hurt to ask. Other options to look into are **internships**, volunteer work, job fairs, and networking events. As we mention in Chapter 5, getting practical experience in the specialty may be difficult – since you're not yet licensed to do anything – but whatever you can do related to neuropsychology, like research work, or volunteering at a hospital or with patient populations (e.g., brain injury, disabled, mentally ill, etc.), can help you make up your mind whether neuropsychology is the career you want to pursue.

Attending a professional conference for one of the national or international neuropsychological organizations can also aid in decision-making. Conferences are fun events, where one can attend lectures on topics of interest, network, and browse or buy books or products related to the subject. Some of the larger organizations in the specialty include the American Psychological Association and, specifically, the Society for Clinical Neuropsychology; the National Academy of Neuropsychology; and the International Neuropsychological Society. Whether you actually attend a live conference or simply read from the websites, you will learn much more about the specialty. If you wish to join, all organizations offer reasonable student rates; each also offers trainee and student resources and ways to get involved, if you choose. Your state or city may also have local or statewide neuropsychological organizations that you can join.

Speak to Others

Once you've narrowed down your choices, you can ask people who know you well their opinions. These may include professors, friends, or relatives. If they are unfamiliar with neuropsychology, you may have to educate them about the subject, but once you've done that you can ask if this is something they can see you doing. If they do know about the specialty, even better; get their input, thoughts, and advice. Some colleges and universities even have mentor services, whereby alumni who are currently working in a career or careers you are interested in can be paired with you, to meet with, shadow, or simply ask questions. In this case, the mentor may not know you personally, but they would be very familiar with the job description and the path it takes to get there. You can also network via LinkedIn and possibly find a mentor that way. Student forums both online and on social media can also be a source of education, support, and advice. Some include the Student Doctor Forum and The Association of Neuropsychology Students in Training (ANST) Facebook Page. You can read previous posts on specific topics or post your own questions. However, keep in mind that all of the above is only other people's opinions. Listen to what others say, but only take it under advisement.

Even this book is meant to expose you to options, demystify the career selection process, and hopefully help with next steps. It alone won't make the decision for you; only you can decide your career path.

References

Bellone, J. A., & Van Patten, R. (2021). *Becoming a neuropsychologist: Advice and guidance for students and trainees.* Springer Nature.

Block, C. (Ed.). (2021). *The neuropsychologist's roadmap: A training and career guide.* American Psychological Association. doi: 10.1037/0000250-000

Bogousslavsky, J., Boller, F., & Iwata, M. (Eds.). (2019). *A history of neuropsychology.* Karger Medical and Scientific Publishers.

Costa, P. T., & McCrae, R. R. (1992). *Revised NEO Personality Inventory (NEO-PI-R) and NEO Five-Factor Inventory (NEO-FFI) Manual.* Psychological Assessment Resources.

Craig, P. (2017) Neuropsychologists. In Sternberg, R. J. *Career paths in psychology: Where your degree can take you.* American Psychological Association.

Furnham, A. (2021). *Twenty ways to assess personnel.* Cambridge University Press. doi: 10.1017/9781108953276

Gati, I., & Asulin-Peretz, L. (2011). Internet-based self-help career assessments and interventions: Challenges and implications for evidence-based career counseling. *Journal of Career Assessment, 19*(3), 259–273.

Holland, J. (1973). *Making vocational choices: A theory of careers*. Prentice-Hall.

Hurtz, G. M., & Donovan, J. J. (2000). Personality and job performance: The Big Five revisited. *Journal of applied psychology, 85*(6), 869.

Kertesz, A. (2006). *The banana lady: And other stories of curious behaviour and speech*. Tafford.

Kolb, B., & Whishaw, I. Q. (2009). *Fundamentals of human neuropsychology*. Macmillan.

Kuther, T. L., & Morgan, R. D. (2019). *Careers in psychology: Opportunities in a changing world*. Sage Publications.

Lezak, M. D., Howieson, D. B., Bigler, E. D. & Tranel, D. (2012). *Neuropsychological assessment* (5th ed.). Oxford University Press.

Loring, D. W., & Bowden, S. (Eds.). (2015). *INS dictionary of neuropsychology and clinical neurosciences*. Oxford University Press, USA.

Morgan, J. E., & Ricker, J. H. (Eds.). (2017). *Textbook of clinical neuropsychology*. Taylor & Francis.

Myers, I. B., McCaulley, M. H., Quenk, N. I., & Hammer, A. L. (2009). *MBTI manual: A guide to the development and use of the Myers-Briggs Type Indicator (3rd ed.)*. CPP, Inc.

Osborn, C. L. (2000). *Over my head: A doctor's own story of head injury from the inside looking out*. Andrews McMeel Publishing.

Pittenger, D. J. (2005). Cautionary comments regarding the Myers-Briggs Type Indicator. *Consulting Psychology Journal: Practice and Research, 57*(3), 210–221. doi: 0.1037/1065–9293.57.3.210

Randall, K., Isaacson, M., & Ciro, C. (2017). Validity and reliability of the Myers-Briggs Personality Type Indicator: A systematic review and meta-analysis. *Journal of Best Practices in Health Professions Diversity, 10*(1), 1–27.

Sacks, O. (2021). *The man who mistook his wife for a hat: And other clinical tales* (Reissue). Vintage (Original work published 1985).

Stein, R., & Swan, A. B. (2019). Evaluating the validity of Myers-Briggs Type Indicator Theory: A teaching tools and window into intuitive psychology. *Social and Personality Psychology Compass, 13*(2), 1–11.

Stromberg, J., & Caswell, E. (2015). Why the Myers-Briggs test is totally meaningless. *Vox*.

Taylor, J. B. (2017). *My stroke of insight: A brain scientist's personal journey*. Viking Adult.

Tieger, P. D., Barron, B., & Tieger, K. (2014). *Do what you are: Discover the perfect career for you through the secrets of personality type*. Hachette UK.

Yang, C., Richard, G., & Durkin, M. (2016). The association between Myers-Briggs Type Indicator and Psychiatry as the specialty choice. *International Journal of Medical Education, 7*, 48–51.

2 Deciding Between Related Career Paths

When narrowing down and choosing a career, there is often some consideration of other, similar careers. It helps to know what these alternative careers do in order to make a decision. Below we will discuss a number of similar occupations to neuropsychology. Websites for the professional organizations mentioned below are included in our book's accompanying eResource.

Neuroscientist

For brain-loving folks who love to do research, a graduate degree (usually a Ph.D.) in neuroscience may be the way to go. Neuroscience is the study of the nervous system, including the brain, and behavioral neuroscience examines the relationship between the nervous system and behavior, cognition, and emotion. The degree itself may be in neurobiology, neurochemistry, computational neuroscience, or something related. Neuroscience programs can be housed in departments of biology, psychology, cognitive science, or as interdisciplinary programs. As a neuroscientist, there are several paths you can take: academia, industry research, consulting, data science, and science journalism, among others (Juavinett, 2020). Even applied areas like marketing, economics, robotics, and artificial intelligence can utilize neuroscience for practical solutions (Freberg, 2022). A neuroscience degree overlaps a great deal with neuropsychology, but typically will not include any clinical training. Therefore, you likely would not be seeing "patients" as part of your job, unless it was strictly for research purposes, and would not have a license to practice. Please see the Society for Neuroscience online for more information. Other, more research-oriented, Ph.Ds. that overlap with neuropsychology include cognitive psychology and experimental psychology.

Medicine

Often, if you are considering neuropsychology, you have probably considered medical school at some point as well. Medical school is very different from

DOI: 10.4324/9781003315513-2

graduate school; training is discussed in more depth elsewhere and is beyond the scope of this book. However, classes in graduate school are smaller, training is often funded, research is a priority, and you don't necessarily graduate with your "class." Coursework is also more theoretical and there is more independent thought. Ph.Ds. increase knowledge in their field by conducting original research. Medical school, by comparison, is a type of professional school, similar to law school, and the curriculum is more standardized. Medical students all take coursework for the first two years in subjects such as anatomy and physiology, epidemiology, microbiology, introduction to clinical medicine, preventative medicine, and different body systems (internal medicine, obstetrics, psych/neuro, pediatrics, surgery). Their third and fourth years are clerkships or clinical rotations in hospitals, in different departments. They do not receive formal training in statistics or research methods in medical school. Interestingly, unlike in psychology, medical students only choose their specialty during their fourth year, when they apply to residencies, and then have to "match" to (hopefully) their choice. Resources to help them do so include books listed in the references of this chapter (Freeman, 2018; Taylor, 2017); see also Student Doctor Network online for more information and an assessment (medical specialty selector) to determine possible medical specialties that best match one's personality and values.

In medicine, there is currently a push for more generalists (primary care, family medicine) since many physicians specialize. Given that you are interested in the brain, however, we will focus on the specialties that deal most with the brain, including psychiatry and neurology (neurosurgery would also apply here, but would obviously involve performing surgery; see *Another Day in the Frontal Lobe* by Katrina Firlik (2006) for a personal account of the neurosurgery field). Psychiatry and neurology historically were one field, which diverged years ago (Paris, 2009). Although their subject matter is similar, even within medicine their training, focus, and day-to-day is different. Both fields, however, can maintain long-term relationships with patients (as opposed to emergency physicians or surgeons). We will also look at the specialty of physiatry, which deals with rehabilitation.

Psychiatrist

Although psychologists and psychiatrists are both doctoral-level professionals that can diagnose and treat mental disorders, their education, training, and what they do on a daily basis are very different. **Psychiatrists** are physicians (medical doctors) and have gone to medical school, their terminal degree being an M.D. or D.O. (Doctor of Osteopathy). They are physicians first. Medical school training is the same whether one ultimately becomes a psychiatrist, a pulmonologist, an oncologist, a surgeon, an emergency room physician, or a pediatrician. As mentioned above, there are classes in all of the body systems, as well as pathology, microbiology, immunology, and pharmacology.

Psychiatrists complete four years of medical school, and then, if they choose psychiatry, complete four years of residency in psychiatry. During residency, they receive didactic and practical training in psychopharmacology, and some programs offer training in psychotherapy (although this is often limited compared to psychologists' training). Psychiatrists focus on mood, psychotic, addictive, behavior, and personality disorders, and treat patients with mental illnesses such as schizophrenia, major depressive disorder, bipolar disorder, or obsessive-compulsive disorder. The psychiatrist obtains a history from the patient and may also request the results of psychological testing, brain imaging, and bloodwork. A psychiatrist can then recommend medication, psychotherapy, further testing, and/or further workup to rule out medical causes that might be contributing to the patient's symptoms. Psychiatrists and (neuro) psychologists often work together and may refer cases to each other. While a psychiatrist may perform a mental status exam or cognitive screener, they will refer to a neuropsychologist for more extensive assessment of cognitive functioning. See the American Psychiatric Association website for more information.

Neurologist

Neurologists also have the prefix "neuro" in their title, indicating the nervous system. **Neurologists** are also licensed and board-certified physicians. The standard examination used by neurologists emphasizes different areas of the nervous system. Neurologists examine more basic functions like sensation, reflexes, and muscle strength, with higher cognitive functions limited to a brief mental status examination. They may see patients with strokes, epilepsy, multiple sclerosis (MS), movement disorders, as well as dementia, but also see patients with headache/migraine, back pain, and problems with the peripheral nervous system. In addition to the physical and neurological exam, neurologists may perform electromyography (EMG) to establish the health of nerves, electroencephalography (EEG) to examine brain waves, may order imaging such as CT or MRI scans, and may perform lumbar punctures ("spinal taps") to examine cerebrospinal fluid. Treatment is of the underlying neurologic disorder via medication. If patients need more thorough cognitive testing, they will be referred to a neuropsychologist. Similarly, if a patient is experiencing problems with mood, affect, or behavior, the neurologist will in turn refer to a psychiatrist and/or psychologist, for medication management and psychotherapy, respectively. Patients with stroke, brain injury, and some movement disorders are also frequently referred to physical rehabilitation, for improvement of functioning and activities of daily living. See the American Neurological Association online for more information.

If you are specifically interested in performing neurodiagnostic tests, there are also careers in **neurodiagnostic technology** (or **surgical neurophysiology**) that do not require a medical degree or a doctorate. Instead, they may require a Bachelor's degree with additional training or a Master's degree. These are healthcare professionals that work under the oversight of a physician (neurologist or surgeon), typically in a hospital and not infrequently in an operating room. They are responsible for intraoperative neuromonitoring during surgery on the brain, spine or nerves, and may also perform EEGs, EMGs and other tests.

Neuropsychiatrist (or Behavioral Neurologist)

In terms of medicine, the closest overlap with neuropsychologists is going to be with **neuropsychiatrists** and **behavioral neurologists**. Neuropsychiatrists are psychiatrists with additional training. Behavioral (or cognitive) neurologists are similar to neuropsychiatrists, but come to the field from neurology, rather than psychiatry. All three professions evaluate and treat injuries and diseases of the brain, and see similar patient populations: those with dementia, brain injury, stroke, seizures, and other neurocognitive disorders. Behavioral neurologists, coming from neurology, focus more on cognitive impairment and aphasia. Neuropsychiatrists focus more on psychiatric, behavioral, and emotional disorders (such as psychosis, **impulsivity**, **abulia**, etc.) arising from neurological injury or illness. Both professions require an additional fellowship in neuropsychiatry/behavioral neurology *after* their residencies in either psychiatry or neurology (or both). Although similar in some ways to neuropsychology, their training is vastly different, as mentioned previously, and these professions perform different activities than neuropsychologists.

Neuropsychiatrists (and behavioral neurologists) conduct a neurological exam and use brief mental status examinations, as psychiatrists and neurologists do, but may also incorporate interview and administer symptom checklists. Although neuropsychiatrists and behavioral neurologists are qualified, by their scope, to administer comprehensive tests of higher cognitive functions, they are much more likely to refer to neuropsychologists to do this. For the amount of time it takes to thoroughly assess higher-order functions, they could see many more patients for medication consultations. Regarding treatment, both neuropsychiatrists and behavioral neurologists utilize medications. Neuropsychiatrists may also do some therapy, but again are more likely to refer out. See the website for the American Neuropsychiatric Association for more information; see also Mendez et al. (1995). As mentioned in Chapter 3, neuropsychologists may provide psychotherapy and/or **cognitive remediation** for treatment and intervention.

Physiatrist

Often confused with the psychiatrist, the "**physiatrist**" is the physician who coordinates physical medicine and rehabilitation. They lead the team of therapists – physical therapists, **occupational therapists**, speech language pathologists, etc. – and others (including social work and psychology) that work with patients recovering from injuries or illnesses including: orthopedic injuries/surgeries, sports injuries, spinal cord injury, MS, amputations, burns, cancer deconditioning, strokes or brain injuries, for example. As physicians, they order tests (bloodwork, imaging), perform some procedures (including EMG and injections), and prescribe medication, physical modalities, and adaptive equipment. Physiatrists take a wholistic, multidisciplinary approach to patient care and improving a patient's functioning, considering not only their musculoskeletal and neurological functioning but also their psychosocial aspects. Physiatrists overlap most with neuropsychologists (and neurologists) when they work primarily with brain injury and stroke, but are medically-oriented physicians that focus more on treatment/rehabilitation than diagnosis (as neurologists do). See the American Academy of Physical Medicine and Rehabilitation website for more about this field and career.

Applied Psychology

As mentioned in Chapter 1, there are both research and applied branches of psychology. Within the applied branches of psychology, there are many different types of psychologists (see also Kuther and Morgan, 2010). The American Psychological Association (APA) recognizes a number of specialties, subspecialties, and proficiencies in professional psychology (American Psychological Association, 2020), some of which we will review briefly here. A **school psychologist**, for example, works within the educational system (often elementary, middle, and high schools) to help children and adolescents with emotional, social, and learning issues. A **counseling psychologist** typically works with less severe types of psychopathologies, may provide vocational counseling, and tends to be employed in university or community counseling centers. A **forensic psychologist** examines individuals who are involved with the legal system and may work within prisons or in court settings. A **clinical psychologist** assesses, diagnoses, and treats more severe forms of mental, emotional, and behavioral issues, and works with patients with anxiety, depression, psychosis, personality disorders, eating disorders, addictions, learning disabilities, and family or relationship issues. As we've discussed, a clinical neuropsychologist is a professional psychologist that has expertise in brain-behavior relationships and uses this knowledge in the assessment, diagnosis, treatment, and/or rehabilitation of those with neurological, medical, developmental, psychiatric, and learning disorders. As you will see, there is a lot of overlap between specialties in what they do. However, ethically, psychologists should always practice within the scope of their competence, via education and specialty training. More information on any specialty can be found on the APA website listed in eResources.

Clinical Psychologist

Unlike psychiatrists, clinical psychologists and other professional psychologists attend graduate school and obtain a doctoral degree in psychology (either a Ph.D. or Psy.D.). Psychology graduate students must also defend a **dissertation** of original research and complete an oral examination to obtain a doctoral degree in most psychology programs. In addition to courses in assessment and psychotherapy, personality, psychopathology, statistics, and experimental methods, graduate students in clinical psychology participate in clinical **externships** (also called **practica**) and an internship. The largest number of applied psychologists are clinical psychologists. Many graduates are generalists, however some also complete **postdoctoral fellowships** in their area of specialty interest (e.g., neuropsychology; geropsychology), typically lasting one to two additional years (as mentioned in Chapter 5). Clinical psychologists are experts in providing psychotherapy and may specialize in specific treatment modalities, such as cognitive behavioral therapy or psychodynamic therapy. They also have training in the administration and interpretation of psychological tests, such as personality tests and intelligence tests. Whereas psychiatrists can prescribe medications in all states, only psychologists who have undergone additional specialized training and education are allowed to prescribe medications and in only a few states at this time (American Psychological Association, 2022).

Rehabilitation Psychologist

Rehabilitation psychologists are professional psychologists with specialized training to work with patients with disabilities and chronic health conditions. They are a small group of applied psychologists (Tackett et al., 2022). They may work in hospitals, rehabilitation facilities, or long-term care facilities and may specialize in working with patients such as amputees, those with brain injury, spinal cord injury, movement disorders, or sensory disabilities (blindness or deafness), to name a few. Many are also involved in research, advocacy, and policy work on behalf of persons with disabilities. While they may overlap with neuropsychologists especially when working with patients with brain injury or stroke, and may also perform cognitive evaluations to inform the rehabilitation team, the rehabilitation psychologist's emphasis *tends* to be more on individual and family therapy and support than assessment.

Clinical Health Psychologist

Clinical health psychologists examine how biological, social, and psychological factors influence health and illness. Clinical health psychology is a specialty that seeks to prevent illness and promote health. Health psychologists may be involved clinically, in research, and/or in designing health policy. They can work in hospitals, specialty clinics, or with agencies or in government. If they see patients, they may work in areas such as: oncology/ cancer, pain management, rehabilitation, medication compliance, drug addiction, obesity and diabetes, heart health, smoking cessation, or sexual health, to provide therapy and education. Therefore, the clinical health psychologist may work with medical patients, like the neuropsychologist does, but diseases/injuries may not have to do with the brain per se. Also, they likely would not be conducting extensive evaluations of cognitive functioning; their assessments are more likely to involve behavioral measures, personality tests, and biopsychosocial measures of factors that affect health outcomes.

Geropsychologist

Older adults are the fastest growing segment of the population, but unfortunately the number of specialists who are trained to work with this group is very small (Moye et al., 2019). **Geropsychologists** specialize in understanding and helping older adults and their families. They can work in hospitals, mental health facilities, private practices, or long-term care facilities. They can also conduct research into health and aging, and do consulting work. Clinically, geropsychologists see older patients for treatment of mental health issues, substance abuse, coping with health issues, dementia and capacity concerns, grief and loss, and end of life care, among other issues. With appropriate training, they may also perform cognitive and functional ability testing, where they overlap with geriatric neuropsychologists.

School Psychologist

As mentioned above, school psychologists work within schools to help children and adolescents with emotional, social, and learning issues. Required training and practice varies somewhat by state, but requires a minimum of "specialist-level" training which includes at least three years of graduate work and a year-long internship. Unless licensed as a psychologist (which requires a doctorate) they cannot practice independently. Some school psychologists do go on for doctoral training. Although school psychologists administer psychological, intelligence, behavioral, and academic/achievement testing to students in a school setting, they traditionally do not receive formal training in neuropsychological tests or have particular expertise in the applied science of brain-behavior relationships. Therefore, they will typically refer a student outside the school to a neuropsychologist for additional neuropsychological testing, if needed. For more information, and guidelines by state, see the website for the National Association of School Psychologists.

For more information about all types of psychologist careers, see The American Psychological Association online. Chapter 5 also discusses psychometrists, who have a Master's degree and certification, and who administer neuropsychological tests but under supervision by a neuropsychologist. They do not interpret test results nor do they work independently.

Other Mental Health Careers

There are other mental health careers that do not entail earning a doctorate, and thus do not take as many years to achieve. However, they do not have the flexibility of allowing for independent assessment, research, and teaching in addition to psychotherapy. Those professionals would also not be able to prescribe medication, like psychiatrists can.

Mental Health Counselor

Mental health counselors (MHC) see patients with anxiety, depression, substance issues, and relationship issues. They are less likely than clinical psychologists to see patients with severe psychopathology. Training varies by state, but typically requires a Master's degree in counseling. See the American Mental Health Counselors Association website for more information.

Marriage and Family Therapists

A **marriage and family therapist** (MFT) assesses, diagnoses, and treats psychological distress within the context of the marriage, couple, and family systems. They may see children and parents, couples, or entire families. MFTs have graduate training (either a Master's or Doctoral degree) in marriage and family therapy and at least two years of clinical experience. See the American Association for Marriage and Family Therapy for more information.

Social Workers

Social workers can be employed in a variety of settings, including hospitals, social service agencies, corporations, criminal justice settings, schools, and private practice. They work with people with mental illnesses and emotional disturbances, marital and family difficulties, substance abuse, behavioral and learning disorders of children and adolescents, or community problems and social issues, depending on their area of specialization. They can provide individual, couples, or group psychotherapy; assist with discharge plans; develop treatment plans; advocate for policy change; and/or identify available resources. Although one can work under supervision with a Bachelor's degree, they require a Master's degree (MSW) for independent practice, although this varies by state. They can also earn a doctorate in Social Work. The National Association of Social Worker has more information on its website.

This is not an exhaustive coverage of careers in mental health. Other careers include, but are not limited to, psychiatric nurses and psychiatric physician assistants (both of whom can also prescribe medications), rehabilitation counselors, substance abuse counselors, and art/music therapists. The Mental Health Professions Career Test (website in eResources) allows you to choose work tasks that you prefer and then provides interest scores for 21 different mental health professions, which may help you include or eliminate certain jobs in your search.

Overall, however, if you prefer a more thorough training in psychotherapy and want the flexibility to engage in testing and research – unique to psychologists over other mental health professionals – psychology may be the better career path for you.

Other Clinical Careers

If your interest in neuropsychology has more to do with working with patients with brain injury, stroke, other neurological illnesses and injuries, and developmental issues, rather than mental health and behavioral concerns per se, other related careers include jobs that you would find in rehabilitation, such as occupational therapy (OT) and speech-language pathology (SLP). Physical therapy could be included here as well, but OT and SLP focus more on cognitive issues and improving a patient's activities of daily living – more similar to neuropsychology – than on ambulation, transfers, and more physical concerns.

Occupational Therapy

Occupational therapists (OTs) help people with disabilities, both by restoring and improving their ability to accomplish daily activities at home and at work and by assisting with accommodations to support accessibility (whether by environmental modifications and/or use of equipment). As part of their assessment, they sometimes do brief evaluations of cognition including memory in addition to evaluation of functional skills. They can work in inpatient or outpatient settings, including hospitals, rehabilitation centers, nursing homes, schools, or for home care agencies. They may see several patients in one day, sometimes more than one at a time. OTs typically have a Master's Degree, depending on the state, although there is currently a movement toward doctoral degrees, such as in physical therapy. OT aides can work with an Associate's or Bachelor's degree, but under supervision. The American Occupational Association has more information on its website.

Speech Language Pathology

Speech and Language Pathologists (SLPs; also called speech therapists) diagnose, evaluate, and treat disorders of speech, voice, swallowing, and/or language. They assess language, overlapping with neuropsychologists, but are often even more comprehensive in this domain. They too may work in inpatient or outpatient settings, including hospitals, rehabilitation centers, nursing homes, schools, or for home care agencies. They can also sometimes be found in private practice or as part of a group practice. Depending on the state, SLPs typically have a graduate degree, either a Master's Degree or a doctorate, in speech language pathology. The website for the American Speech-Language-Hearing Association contains more information.

Although both OTs and SLPs can see similar patients to neuropsychologists, and may engage the patients in cognitive remediation (see Chapter 3), their scope of practice and training does not include performing any psychotherapy. Similarly, while they may do brief assessments of memory or language, their assessments are not comprehensive evaluations of the entirety of cognition or of mood. Both professions are also less likely to teach or perform independent research, unless they have doctorates in their field.

As we mentioned in Chapter 1, part of choosing a career is considering other, similar and overlapping careers. The above careers in research (neuroscience) and clinical fields of medicine (psychiatry, neurology, neuropsychiatry/behavioral neurology, physiatry), applied psychology, mental health, and rehabilitation all share many of the same interests as neuropsychologists. Clinically, they may all see similar patients, and often work with and refer to each other. However, their training, the skills they utilize, and their day-to-day routines all vary quite considerably. The personalities and work values of people in these careers may be different than for neuropsychologists as well. However, we hope that a review and exploration of the similarities and differences of some of the more common overlapping careers can help you narrow down your possibilities and assist with your career decision-making. Even if you ultimately do not decide on neuropsychology for a career, we want you to choose the best fit for you!

References

American Psychological Association (2020, October). *Recognized specialties, sub-specialties, and proficiencies in professional psychology.* https://www.apa.org/ed/graduate/specialize/recognized

American Psychological Association (2022, January). *About prescribing psychologists.* https://www.apaservices.org/practice/advocacy/authority/prescribing-psychologists

Firlik, K. (2006). *Another day in the frontal lobe: A brain surgeon exposes life on the inside.* Random House.

Freberg, L. (2022). *An introduction to applied behavioral neuroscience: Biological psychology in everyday life.* Taylor & Francis.

Freeman, B. S. (2018). *The ultimate guide to choosing a medical specialty* (4th ed.). McGraw-Hill.

Juavinett, A. (2020). *So you want to be a neuroscientist?* Columbia University Press.

Kuther, T. L., & Morgan, R. D. (2019). *Careers in psychology: Opportunities in a changing world.* Sage Publications.

Mendez, M. F., Van Gorp, W., & Cummings, J. L. (1995). Neuropsychiatry, neuropsychology, and behavioral neurology: A critical comparison. *Cognitive and Behavioral Neurology, 8*(4), 297–302.

Moye, J., Karel, M. J., Stamm, K. E., Qualls, S. H., Segal, D. L., Tazeau, Y. N., & Di-Gilio, D. A. (2019). Workforce analysis of psychological practice with older adults: Growing crisis requires urgent action. *Training and Education in Professional Psychology, 13*(1), 46.

Paris, J. (2009). Psychiatry and neuroscience. *The Canadian Journal of Psychiatry, 54*(8), 513–517.

Tackett, M. J., Gorgens, K., Miller, M. A., & Lyman, K. H. (2022). Understanding the rehabilitation psychology specialty career pathway. *Rehabilitation Psychology, 67*(1), 1.

Taylor, A. (2017). *How to choose a medical specialty* (6th ed.). Student Doctor Network.

3 What Do Neuropsychologists Do and Where Are They Found?

Now that you know a little more about the specialty of neuropsychology and similarities and differences between neuropsychology and related professions, it is helpful to know where neuropsychologists can work and what their day-to-day activities are like in each setting. As you will see in this chapter, the profession of neuropsychology is a very flexible one, and a neuropsychologist can work in various kinds of settings depending on their interests, career path, and lifestyle (Craig, 2017). Many have very active careers and work in more than one of these areas too! A recent survey of all neuropsychologists across the country showed that of the people who responded, about 84% work full time, 8% work part time, and 7% have both full and part-time jobs (Sweet et al., 2021). Neuropsychology is also an adaptable specialty that can easily grow in different directions as needs in different settings change over time. According to the survey by Sweet and others (2021), neuropsychologists as a group are very satisfied with their jobs. Job satisfaction for neuropsychologists ranged from ratings of 76 to 85 out of 100, with those in private practice reporting more satisfaction; those in multiple work settings had slightly lower satisfaction. Income satisfaction was the same across settings, in the mid-70s.

The main thing that all neuropsychologists have in common is that they are all trained to administer, score, understand, interpret, and share the results of **standardized tests** that evaluate different kinds of cognitive problems (Craig, 2017). As noted in a previous chapter, "cognition" is another word for "thinking skills," and many brain-related diagnoses have distinct patterns of cognitive strengths and difficulties that can be identified using these tests. Different aspects of cognition are associated with different areas and pathways within the brain that are impacted by various illnesses or injuries. Neuropsychologists are trained to know which cognitive patterns fit with which diagnoses, especially in the areas in which they specialize. For example, people with Alzheimer's disease tend to score lower on memory tests and people with Parkinson's disease may score lower on timed tests and tests that involve understanding information that they visually perceive. This information can then be used

DOI: 10.4324/9781003315513-3

to help figure out a correct diagnosis, identify a person's areas of cognitive strength and difficulty, and better understand a person's abilities, behaviors, and likely course of and response to treatment (Harvey, 2022). Testing can also be performed as a baseline, such as before surgery. Chapter 4 of this book provides descriptions of the different kinds of patients that neuropsychologists may work with from early childhood through older adult, and what kinds of diagnoses they tend to see.

A standardized test is one that is given to many test subjects as it is being developed. It is administered to everyone in exactly the same way, so that it is known how people generally tend to perform and what might be considered a higher or lower than typical score. Tests of Intelligence Quotient (IQ) are standardized tests, for instance, and help to measure where a gifted student may have areas of strength or where a student with a learning disability may be struggling. Neuropsychologists may use parts of IQ tests or tests that are similar to IQ tests to measure the cognitive aspects of different brain diseases in the settings where they work. This information is often used to help with treatment planning in clinical settings and may be used for research studies too.

Neuropsychologists often see patients for a few hours for assessment, either all at once or broken up over a few visits. Children are often assessed in one session (to prevent missing multiple days of school), as are some older adults who may not have the stamina for long or multiple testing sessions. The assessment visit(s) include a review of their medical records and a thorough interview, asking them (and any family that may attend) about the patient's symptoms and their history. Then the neuropsychologist chooses the paper-pencil tests, and perhaps some that are computer-administered, that will best answer the referral question. The reason testing takes time is because neuropsychologists are testing many different cognitive domains, such as attention, memory, language, visuospatial functions, executive functioning, mood and sometimes personality. Also, memory is assessed over time, in order to examine both short-term, or immediate, memory and then long-term memory. This extends the amount of time it takes with the patient.

In addition to testing, neuropsychologists can also provide treatment. If they have the relevant training, they may be able to provide a specialized treatment called "cognitive remediation" (Parente & Stapleton, 1997; Sohlberg & Mateer, 2001; Prigatano, 2005; Kirsch-Darrow & Tsao, 2021), where they can help patients improve their memory, organization, or other areas where the tests show that they are having cognitive difficulty. The goals of this treatment are often to help patients perform functionally better in their everyday life, such as to remember to take their medication, come to their appointments, or remember plans with their friends. Depending on their training and the setting where they work, neuropsychologists can also provide more traditional psychotherapy and/or group therapy. The emotional, behavioral, and interpersonal effects of brain injury and other neurological illness can be extremely disturbing for the patient as well as the family, and can affect the ability of the individual to live independently. However, psychotherapy with patients that have suffered brain injury or other neurological illnesses that affect their thinking is adapted specifically for this population, as these patients often have difficulties with awareness and acceptance due to their organic illness and may also suffer from behavioral disturbances as a result (Klonoff, 2010; Ruff & Chester, 2014). Finally, providing feedback to the patient about their testing results can also be therapeutic (Postal & Armstrong 2013), particularly if ongoing consultation is offered afterward. The advantage to doing both assessment and treatment with different patients is the balance between more short-term relationships (assessment) and longer-term relationships (treatment), although it is not uncommon for someone to be re-tested later.

Another set of tools for neuropsychologists that work in comprehensive epilepsy center settings is in performing pre- and post-surgical testing, as well as specialized surgical Wada procedures (see example under *Academic Medicine* below), electrocortical mapping, and/or functional imaging (Morrison et al., 2018). Training for these procedures can be obtained at the postdoctoral level for those who wish to work in this area.

The subsections below illustrate what the work is like for neuropsychologists, and other professionals with neuropsychology backgrounds, who work in various (although not all possible) settings. Unique to this book are quotes from actual neuropsychologists about what their day-to-day is like.

Clinical versus Research

Many neuropsychologists work primarily in clinical settings where they evaluate people with standardized test batteries to figure out how to help them get better, and some neuropsychologists do research by writing grants, conducting studies, publishing the results of these studies, and giving lectures about the aspects of the brain on which they do research. Depending on the setting, some neuropsychologists do a combination of both clinical work and research (Grote et al., 2016). Research is often conducted at private facilities, government agencies, and at academic institutions. A description of the more clinical settings is provided below, but first here is what a typical day is like for two neuropsychologists who (also) do research:

> I remember being told, "You can't do research AND clinical care," and I'm glad I didn't listen. As a clinician, I conduct neuropsychological evaluations and neurocognitive interventions with patients with traumatic brain injury (TBI) or other acquired neurological disorders – my clinical work has always informed my research. As Director of the Brain Injury Research Center at a large academic medical center, I lead a team of faculty, staff, fellows, and students who are interested in understanding clinical and biological sequelae of TBI, including post-traumatic neurodegeneration.

Our Center has a longstanding commitment to developing and validating neurobehavioral treatments for TBI survivors, so we also conduct clinical trials of novel interventions. I spend a lot of my days in meetings with my team, and with colleagues across the world, as our research is inherently interdisciplinary and highly collaborative. We discuss logistics of study implementation, train staff members on new protocols, brainstorm ways to overcome logistical barriers, analyze and review data, and develop manuscripts and presentations to share our results. On any given day, I may meet with neuroradiologists, neuropathologists, therapists, neurologists, neurosurgeons, physiatrists, biostatisticians, epidemiologists, and implementation scientists. I learn something new every day.

Kristen Dams-O'Connor, Ph.D.

As Deputy Director of an institute at the National Institutes of Health, there is no typical day. From working with the leadership of our intramural research laboratories and our extramural grant programs on our scientific priorities, to reviewing new federal rules or regulations that impact our funding, or planning the scientific strategy for the institute as a whole, I am asked to move seamlessly between a number of scientific topics and areas. I also work with the leadership at NIH and at the Department of Health and Human Services on multiple strategic groups that involve our scientific areas, such as maternal health, reproductive health, and disability, or on groups that involve advancing the science in patient-centered outcomes or scientific data sharing. As a supervisor, I work with a range of professionals in communications, science policy, legislation and public policy, data science, global health, and health equity to ensure we are leading our scientific programs in line with our Congressional language, meeting the needs of our stakeholders, and advancing diversity, equity, inclusion, and accessibility in all aspects of our work. Finally, I work with scientists across the nation and around the world, as well as patient and provider advocacy groups to ensure that the science we do ultimately advances our vision of "Healthy Pregnancies. Healthy Children. Healthy and Optimal Lives."

Alison N. Cernich, Ph.D., ABPP-CN

Hospital Settings

Many neuropsychologists work in hospital settings, including community hospitals, large academic medical centers, psychiatric hospitals, and through the Veteran's Health Administration (VA hospitals). Some independent centers even specialize in a particular disorder, such as epilepsy centers, memory disorder centers, or cancer care centers, and neuropsychologists can be found there as well. In most hospital settings, evaluations conducted by a neuropsychologist are shared with treatment team members who are working with the same patient in different ways, including one or more physicians as well as people from related professions described in Chapter 2. In each of these settings the neuropsychologist uses standardized tests to evaluate the different kinds of brain-related diagnoses that their patients have, and makes recommendations for treatment based on how the patient performs. In a community hospital, for instance, a neuropsychologist may provide brief screenings to assess for overall level of cognitive function when a patient presents with any number of medical diagnoses that have direct or indirect effects on the brain, as well as various psychiatric disorders.

Academic Medicine

Academic medical centers are often large, dynamic environments where the neuropsychologist may have opportunities to work in more specialized programs that focus on areas like child development, epilepsy, memory disorders, multiple sclerosis, stroke, Parkinson's disease, traumatic brain injury, rehabilitation, schizophrenia, bipolar disorder, or addiction (described further in Chapter 4). These programs can be housed in departments of Neurology, Psychiatry, Rehabilitation Medicine, Pediatrics, Geriatrics, Neurosurgery, or other departments in the medical center. Often these programs have strong research components within them, as well as connections to various training programs where medical students, psychology students, and/or students of nursing, social work, occupational therapy, physical therapy, speech and language pathology, and other healthcare trainees may come to learn (Bellone & Van Patten, 2021). A neuropsychologist may play a role in the training process of any or all of these disciplines. Academic medical centers also offer opportunities for ongoing education for all professionals, including neuropsychologists, such as lectures by visiting professors on a variety of topics (i.e., **"Grand Rounds"**).

In my role as Director of Neuropsychology Service in the department of Neurology at an academic hospital, I see patients presenting with questions about their brain functioning, conduct clinical research, and have opportunities to teach graduate students in psychology, as well as medical residents and fellows. Patients in my practice include those with epilepsy, dementia, and brain injury, and through conducting neuropsychological evaluations I obtain unique information about their cognition, intellect, and psychological symptoms. I routinely interact with neurologists and psychiatrists and work with neurosurgeons and neuro-interventional radiologists when patients are undergoing Wada testing, whereby a medication is injected to temporarily "put the brain to sleep" on one side (or hemisphere) at a time, while I test language and memory abilities on the other side. As a scientist-practitioner, I collaborate in research which informs my work with patients, and I attend conferences to present my research and to continue learning from my colleagues. Much of my time outside of these activities is devoted to going over the test data, writing reports to document the neuropsychological findings, and to supervising students who are training to be neuropsychologists.

Luba Nakhutina, Ph.D., ABPP-CN

As a Director of Pediatric Neuropsychology, with clinical, administrative, and training roles, no day is EVER the same! Two–three days per week, a trainee and I administer comprehensive neuropsychological evaluations to children/adolescents from toddler ages through young adulthood. Our clinical neuropsychology division is part of the neurology department, so I evaluate children with a range of neurological disorders, such as acquired conditions (brain injuries, stroke, brain tumors) and congenital diagnoses (spina bifida, cerebral palsy, Down syndrome). On my non-clinical days, I provide supervision to trainees (externs, interns, and postdoctoral fellows), and participate in lots of meetings for administrative obligations, including: as Assistant Chair of the organization's Psychology Committee, Co-Chair of the Psychology Continuing Education (CE) committee, member of the hospital's Credentials Committee, and on the Board of Directors for my state's neuropsychology organization. I also spend several hours per week writing and editing neuropsychological reports and responding to messages from colleagues and families/patients. Throughout the year, I provide lectures for our neuropsychology didactic series, present at a Grand Rounds or professional conference, and write or review scholarly publications. I am fortunate to be quite efficient and a great advocate for myself, so I never work in the evenings or on weekends.

Gianna Locascio, Psy.D., ABPP

Psychiatric Settings

Neuropsychologists at state and other psychiatric hospitals, or in Psychiatry Departments in medical centers, work with individuals who have more serious mental illnesses, including schizophrenia and bipolar disorder. They may do evaluations to help the treatment team better understand a patient's cognitive difficulties in order to decide how to best help them in these areas. In state hospitals with a forensic component, the information the neuropsychologist collects through the testing battery may also be used for legal decision-making, for instance deciding on a patient's ability to understand the nature of a crime that they have allegedly committed.

I am a licensed clinical psychologist in the Department of Psychiatry in an academic medical center. My work, which focuses on the evaluation and treatment of cognitive health in people with serious mental illness, is carried out in many forms. Within the domain of research, I have developed and led clinical trials to test the efficacy and effectiveness of cognitive remediation to address the cognitive impairment associated with schizophrenia. The ultimate purpose of this research is to inform the implementation of scalable, evidence-based practices to support individuals' recovery and functioning in the community. I have applied the knowledge gained through research to develop a service model to assess and address cognitive health needs within community-based mental health programs, and provide training and supervision to other mental health professionals to support its implementation. These collective experiences inform my own delivery of skills training interventions as a practitioner in a clinical care setting which, in turn, yields new perspectives on what further research is needed to optimize cognition and recovery among people with serious mental illness.

Alice M. Saperstein, Ph.D.

Veterans Affairs (VA) Hospitals

Neuropsychologists who work at Veterans Affairs (VA) hospitals focus on work with veterans and their families. Some veterans have been in combat and some have not, but all have shared unique experiences that often cause them to form special connections with each other. Although veterans may experience many similar medical and psychiatric conditions to those of civilians, those that have been in combat also have experienced unique circumstances surrounding their problems that need to be addressed by neuropsychologists with specialization in this area. Veterans who suffered a traumatic brain injury in a war, for instance, may also have other serious physical injuries as well as depression, anxiety, Posttraumatic Stress Disorder, and even addiction as a result of trauma from the war.

As a neuropsychologist in a VA hospital, I have the opportunity to provide clinical services in a variety of settings, to work with interprofessional colleagues on various teams, and to be involved in psychology training, staff development, and quality improvement and systems change. A typical day for me might look like the following: I begin the day meeting with my postdoctoral trainee who reviews and prepares to see a neuropsychology consult that morning (a 72 y.o. veteran, exposed to Agent Orange in the Vietnam war and reporting some changes in language functioning). While the postdoc is completing the consultation including interview and administration of tests, I am available to step into the consultation to meet the patient and family member, and consult with the postdoc about additional tests. That morning, I also work on preparing for a presentation I am making the following day at the primary care team's meeting to review the pilot project we are rolling out to improve our detection of patients with undetected dementia diagnoses. In the afternoon, I meet with my postdoctoral training committee to plan our upcoming interviews for the next training year. Then I have a virtual psychotherapy session with a veteran, who is caregiving for his wife with Alzheimer's disease, to provide an evidence-based treatment for caregivers of dementia patients. Later in the afternoon, I run a group in our geriatric primary care clinic for veterans with mild cognitive impairment. The end of the day is a combination of catching up on chart notes, emailing with other providers about a case we will be discussing tomorrow, and returning some phone calls. I leave at the end of the day feeling a sense of accomplishment and looking forward to tomorrow.

Valerie Abel, Psy.D., ABPP

Rehabilitation Centers

There are two kinds of places that people often think of when they think of rehabilitation centers: the kind where people go to recover from a problem with alcohol or drugs and the kind where people go to recover from an injury or illness that affected the brain, including stroke, traumatic brain injury, or a brain tumor. Either kind of rehabilitation center can be connected to a hospital or be a freestanding program, and neuropsychologists can work in either one. In rehabilitation centers focused on brain injury or illness, neuropsychologists play the important role of evaluating patients to clarify the cognitive difficulties a person has as a result of the problem that brought them into rehabilitation. Similar to hospital settings, they work as part of a team including a physician as well as physical therapists, speech therapists, and occupational therapists. The information they collect in their evaluations can be used to help the whole treatment team work with a patient; for instance, it may be best for the patient to take notes in all of their therapies if they are having problems with memory and forgetting to do their home exercises in between sessions. In a rehabilitation setting, cognitive rehabilitation can help the patients with their areas of cognitive difficulty and/or individual or group therapy can help them cope with and adjust to what has happened to them (Bellone & Van Patten, 2021). Assessment can help determine whether treatment has been effective (van Heugten et al., 2020).

As Director of Psychology Research at a university-based rehabilitation hospital, my daily activities include clinical research, supervising post-doctoral psychology students, ensuring compliance with institutional and federal regulations for protection of human subjects, other administrative tasks such as budgets and employee evaluations, and providing psychological services directly to patients. As a rehabilitation psychologist, my focus is on the adjustment of people living with chronic health conditions and disabilities. Because I work primarily with people with neurological conditions such as brain injury or stroke, I typically use test data from cognitive assessments – similar to those used by neuropsychologists – in order to enhance adjustment to disability and improve everyday functioning.

The treatment process may involve individual and group psychotherapy, as well as remedial interventions focused on improving positive cognitive abilities such as problem-solving skills. On any given day, I might meet with patients or research participants, supervise postdoctoral students on their research and clinical work, review manuscripts submitted for publication in scientific journals, write my own research papers or book chapters, attend administrative meetings, and consult with multidisciplinary research teams preparing grant applications for funding.

Joseph Rath, Ph.D.

Nursing Homes

Because people in nursing homes are typically older, they are more likely to have conditions such as Alzheimer's disease or other medical conditions that can impact the brain and cause cognitive difficulties that make it more difficult for them to take care of themselves. A primary role of neuropsychologists in nursing homes may be to administer brief cognitive evaluations to track whether nursing home residents are showing decline in cognitive function. This information can be used by the team to help them decide how much structure and support a nursing home resident may need and other such decisions. Similar to their role in rehabilitation centers, neuropsychologists who work in nursing homes may also offer cognitive interventions and/or individual or group psychotherapy for the residents.

Neuropsychologists provide services to residents of long-term care and skilled nursing facility centers in a comprehensive manner. They are actively engaged in assessment, in intervention, in teaching / supervising, and consulting with other healthcare professionals. They assess and treat individuals with dementia so that residents can have a better quality of life for a longer period of time. Neuropsychologists often treat such major problems as anxiety, depression, adjustment disorders, psychosis, and behavior disturbances. In addition, they offer invaluable information to the team of professionals regarding the design of behavioral interventions for medical problems as non-compliance. During the onset of the pandemic, neuropsychologists in long-term care facilities were among the first among clinical providers to observe and document the long-haul cognitive and psychiatric sequelae of COVID-19.

Kristine T. Kingsley, PsyD, ABPP

Private Practice

Many neuropsychologists work in private practices, either as their primary setting or part-time in addition to one or more of the other settings described in this chapter. In fact, the survey of neuropsychologists noted above showed that about 55% worked in a setting such as a hospital or rehabilitation center only, 24% were in private practice only, and 21% worked in both private practice and in another setting (Sweet et al., 2021).

A main difference between a private practice and work in a hospital setting is that in a private practice, the neuropsychologist typically works either on their own or within a group practice of other psychologists and/or neuropsychologists, but not as often with a treatment team made up of other disciplines (Bellone & Van Patten, 2021). A benefit of a private practice is that the neuropsychologist can set their own hours and work as much or as little as they would like. Payment scales are also set by the neuropsychologist, so compared to a hospital setting there is a much wider range of income that a neuropsychologist in a private practice can make. A private practice is a business, however, and the neuropsychologist is responsible for what is called "overhead," meaning that they must pay for their own rent and supplies, including the tests that they give, whereas this is already covered in a hospital setting. They are also less limited in terms of taking time off, but this vacation time (as well as sick time) is unpaid. Neuropsychologists in a private practice must also have their own insurance policies (i.e., health insurance, malpractice), whereas this is typically provided to neuropsychologists in a hospital setting. Some people may feel isolated in a private practice setting, particularly if they work completely solo and not part of a group practice, and there is less opportunity for interdisciplinary consultation or collaboration (thus, it is important to "know yourself" - see Chapter 1). In addition, a neuropsychologist in private practice is responsible for their own record keeping and has less direct oversight for this than one in a hospital setting might. Finally, as private practices typically don't have supports for conducting research, including medical library access, these opportunities are more limited in this kind of setting (Pepping, 2015).

As is the case for most neuropsychologists, neuropsychologists in private practice are typically members of both local and national organizations such as the American Academy of Clinical Neuropsychology (AACN), the American Psychological Association (APA), the International Neuropsychological Society (INS), and the National Academy of Neuropsychology (NAN). Membership in these organizations offers many services to support neuropsychologists in private practice who may have less daily contact with colleagues. One example is the APA Office of Legal and Regulatory Affairs, which can provide advice to neuropsychologists in areas such as starting a new practice, record keeping, legal issues, and audits by insurance companies (American Psychological Association, 2019). The AACN offers several listservs or email lists where neuropsychologists from around the country can consult with one another on a variety of practice-related topics (see link in eResources). A more complete description of other similar listservs can be found through the Society of Clinical Neuropsychology.

Clinically, a neuropsychologist in private practice is free to build their own practice entirely in line with their own interests and areas of expertise. They can focus on any population described in Chapter 4 as long as they have had the right training in this area. Most states also require a certain number of **Continuing Education (CE)** credits for neuropsychologists to keep their licenses to practice (Custom Continuing Education, LLC., n.d.). These CE credits are relevant to all psychologists and neuropsychologists, but may be even more helpful for those in private practice who may not have as much direct access to educational opportunities to ensure their knowledge stays up-to-date.

Here are some examples of what some neuropsychologists in private practice do day-to-day:

I am a founding partner of our 20-year-old group practice of neuropsychologists, clinical psychologists, and rehabilitation specialists. My week is a balancing act between being a clinician, overseeing our group practice, currently being president of the New York State Association of Neuropsychology, and being a mom of three teenage boys. A "typical" week (if nothing unexpected comes up but it always does) consists of remote interviews on Mondays, report writing on Tuesdays, neuropsychological evaluations on Wednesdays and Fridays, and remote feedbacks and group practice meetings on Thursdays. Mixed among those days is always more report writing, committee meetings, advocating for patients, overseeing billing and insurance issues, being available to consultants in our practice, keeping up on the research and clinical literature, consulting and testifying for legal cases, attending CSE meeting for students, managing NYSAN tasks, responding to patient questions, and submitting billing. As a college student, I would never have imagined being in such a position. It would have intimidated me. It is only with time and experience that such a full and rewarding life can be developed.

Cindy L. Breitman, Ph.D., ABPP-CN

As a solo private practitioner, I have been able to purposefully schedule my work weeks with a large variety of patients and activities, which keeps the job interesting. I appreciate controlling my own schedule, deciding which patient populations I aim to serve, and having the flexibility to specialize in clinical areas that are of particular interest to me. Along the way, I have learned how to own and operate a successful business, including how to manage patient flow, perform corporate accounting, and navigate the world of healthcare insurance. In addition to conducting neuropsychological assessments and providing psychotherapy services across the lifespan, I also work as an adjunct professor at a local university to provide supervision to students completing their doctorate degrees in clinical psychology. It is rewarding to share my accumulated knowledge and experience with those just entering the field as a way to both influence and give back to the profession.

Linda S. LaMarca, Ph.D., ABPP-CN

Teaching

Some neuropsychologists work primarily as professors, most commonly in Departments of Psychology in university settings (Bellone & Van Patten, 2021). These neuropsychologists may teach only at one level, for instance undergraduate, or they may teach a combination of courses at the undergraduate, Master's, and/or doctoral levels. Sometimes they can even teach courses within other departments, such as in Departments of Biology or Neuroscience. A neuropsychologist is likely to focus on courses related to cognitive psychology, physiological psychology, and/or abnormal psychology, but depending on the university and the size of the faculty he or she may also teach courses including the history of psychology, experimental psychology, or developmental psychology. These courses are generally conducted through the academic year, from September through May. In addition to teaching, neuropsychologists in university settings play important roles in mentoring students and are frequently part of Master's Degree thesis and doctoral dissertation committees.

Often, neuropsychologists who work in university settings also have their own research labs. They commonly write grants to help fund their research. Many times, they are able to pay graduate students to help in their lab, and undergraduate students may also have opportunities to gain experience in this kind of lab setting. In addition to their universities, neuropsychologists who have labs may be connected to hospitals or other clinical settings where they can recruit people with various brain-related diagnoses to participate in their studies. Although their teaching takes place during the academic year, their lab work may be year-round.

As a core faculty member in a clinical psychology doctoral program, my primary responsibilities are teaching courses (e.g., research methods, the neuroanatomical and neurophysiological foundation of neuropsychology, clinical psychopharmacology, and assessment practicum) and supporting the students on my research team in the development and completion of their dissertation projects. Additionally, I am involved in conducting research and sharing the results with the scientific community and the general public through presentations, training materials, and published manuscripts. One unique aspect of our doctoral program is the fact that it is housed in a bilingual (American Sign Language: ASL and English) and multicultural university for undergraduate and graduate students who are Deaf, DeafBlind, and hard of hearing. In light of this fact, I navigate various languages (e.g., ASL, Tactile ASL, English) and communication modalities throughout the day, and also am frequently engaged in discussions about training, research, ethical issues and professional practice involving people from different cultures and who hold intersectional identities. Outside of this work, I have a small private practice providing neuropsychological assessments to individuals across the lifespan who are Deaf, hard of hearing, DeafBlind, and blind/low vision, as well as clinical supervision and consultation services to hearing neuropsychologists working with clients from these communities.

Lawrence Pick, Ph.D., ABPP-CN

I would call myself a "generalist" neuropsychologist because I practice neuropsychology in a variety of settings, including as an adjunct professor, in the foster care system, and in early intervention. I teach undergraduate and graduate students and supervise first year clinical students in assessment. I incorporate neuropsychology into all my courses so students can understand how brain-behavior relationships inform knowledge in the undergraduate psychology curriculum. As an adjunct professor in a college specializing in forensic psychology and criminal justice, I introduce neuropsychological concepts in all courses from developmental psychology to the psychology of criminal behavior. An understanding of neuropsychology has become especially important in analyzing the critical issues involving the development of the frontal lobe in adolescents and its impact on the legal issues surrounding the death penalty and life incarceration for adolescents and young people in the United States. Further, many clients in our mental health clinics and community settings, including foster care and domestic violence centers, have a history of brain injuries, concussions, diseases that affect the brain, and falls that are the consequence of alcoholism and substance abuse. It is important to be knowledgeable about the neuropsychological history of these special client groups who are often from underserved communities and are people of color.

Bridget Amatore, Ph.D.

Forensic Settings

According to the American Board of Professional Psychology, forensic psychology is the "application of the science and profession of psychology to questions and issues relating to law and the legal system" (American Board of Professional Psychology, 2023). There are a range of settings that are considered forensic, as described below. A neuropsychologist who has had the additional forensic training and experience, a **forensic neuropsychologist**, brings a unique specialty to these settings as he or she is able to apply standardized tests of cognition to answer questions that are related to the legal and/or the treatment aspects of the cases.

Courts

A neuropsychologist may conduct interviews and/or standardized assessments for the courts for a variety of reasons. A neuropsychologist working for a family court, for instance, may conduct cognitive assessments to be included in court records in the context of custody evaluations. They may also interview someone who is alleged to be incapacitated (Schaefer & Farrer, 2022), in addition to other interested parties, and report their findings to the court in a guardianship hearing. Neuropsychologists who work for the courts are often asked to testify as expert witnesses based on the findings of their evaluations.

Forensic Hospitals

Neuropsychologists who work in forensic hospitals typically work with clients who have serious mental illness and/or problems with drugs or alcohol in addition to legal charges; these clients may be at different stages of the legal process. The neuropsychologist may work on a pre-trial unit, where individuals have recently been charged with criminal acts but have not yet gone through the legal system because of how their mental illness has impacted their ability to understand the charges against them and/or to be able to participate in the legal process. One role of a neuropsychologist in this kind of unit is to help assess an individual's legal competence in these areas.

On a post-trial unit, the neuropsychologist works with individuals who have already been through the legal process and it has been determined by the court that because of their mental illness, the individual did not understand the wrongful nature of the crime they committed and/or couldn't participate meaningfully in their defense. People in this situation are acquitted as "Not Guilty by Reason of Insanity (NGRI)," and although they don't serve a legal sentence, they are often required to receive long-term mental health care. A neuropsychologist on a post-trial unit may conduct neuropsychological evaluations with these individuals for treatment purposes or to help decide when they can be moved to a level of care that has a different level of restrictions and structure.

Correctional Settings

Neuropsychologists may also work with people who are in jail or who have been sentenced to prison in local, state, or federal facilities. Similar to people in forensic hospitals because of a crime that they committed, inmates in prison may suffer from mental illness, physical illness, and/or addiction, but these individuals have been legally convicted of and sentenced for their crime and have not been acquitted on a NGRI plea. A neuropsychologist's role is similar across correctional settings; they use standardized cognitive tests to help decide an inmate's competency to stand trial or their level of understanding of the crime of which they are being accused. These tests can also be used to help decide about treatment planning, transfer to a different level of structure, and/or whether it is safe to release an inmate into the community once they have completed a sentence. Like neuropsychologists in other settings, those who work in jails or prisons typically work with an interdisciplinary team. They also may be called as an expert witness to present the findings of their evaluation to the court.

Independent Medical Examinations

Sometimes a court would like to hear the opinion of an independent neuropsychologist in making legal decisions, in addition to or instead of one who is already affiliated with the legal system. In these instances, a lawyer may call upon a neuropsychologist who is in private practice to conduct an evaluation called an Independent Medical Examination (IME), where the neuropsychologist uses standardized cognitive tests to answer similar questions about whether the person being accused of a crime can understand their responsibility or whether a victim of an alleged crime has suffered from cognitive problems as a result. Examples of cases involving a victim may include decisions related to whether the victim now has cognitive problems related to a head injury after an assault (personal injury case), or medical malpractice cases where a victim may have cognitive problems because of a mistake allegedly made by a physician or hospital. Neuropsychologists can also make recommendations as to whether someone is disabled and should receive insurance benefits, for example after suffering a stroke.

Here are work descriptions from two neuropsychologists who focus on forensics:

> Following my training in neuropsychology I took a job at a forensic state psychiatric hospital where I learned to apply neuropsychological principles to the issues of dangerousness, criminal responsibility and competency to stand trial. The work involved developing and adding forensic opinions to the evaluative process. An important part of the process was learning how to detect poor effort and malingering of both cognitive and psychiatric disorders, as well as how to give testimony and depositions as an expert witness. Over time, I began to do this work in a private practice setting and expanded it to include the areas of aid in sentencing, child custody, guardianship, civil commitment, disability, independent medical/ neuropsychological examinations and personal injury lawsuits. In contrast to clinical evaluations, the person being evaluated is not a "patient" and may not have control over access to the results – reports are written for 3rd parties (attorneys, judges, insurance companies, employers).
>
> Sid Binks, Ph.D., ABPP-CN

> As the founder of my private practice, which primarily focuses on forensic, forensic neuropsychological, and clinical neuropsychological evaluations and consultation, I get a chance to wear many hats!

Although there are certain activities that I tend to do each week (e.g., speaking to attorneys, administering and scoring tests, writing reports), the specific tasks and schedule of each day are different. My work is comprised of running the business of my practice, as well as managing/performing the evaluation and consultation work, teaching (I work with both predoctoral and postdoctoral trainees and am an adjunct professor in a graduate program at a local university), and being engaged in local and national professional organizations in both forensic and neuropsychology.

Specific to my forensic work, I conduct both criminal and civil forensic neuropsychological evaluations (e.g., adjudicative competence, mitigation, testamentary capacity, and independent medical evaluations, or IMEs). The majority of my criminal evaluations are conducted at a prison or at a local hospital, where the examinee is brought from the jail to a forensic unit of the hospital which can offer private interview rooms. The rest of my criminal and civil forensic evaluations, as well as my clinical and consultative work, is performed at either the office of an attorney or my own, at a courthouse, or remotely via a videoconferencing platform. Finally, I absolutely love teaching whether it is at the university, a medical center, in my practice, or at a conference, as I get to learn at the same time! I feel incredibly lucky that there is so much diversity in what I do and with whom I get the privilege to work.

Chriscelyn Tussey, Psy.D., ABPP

Industry

Sometimes neuropsychologists work in less traditional settings where they primarily do research in different areas for larger companies. Two examples of this are in the areas of test development and pharmaceutical research. In test development, the neuropsychologist either works for the companies that make the tests and measures or attains independent funding to create the tests and measures that other neuropsychologists then use clinically in any of the settings described above. Neuropsychologists can also work in pharmaceuticals for drug companies and help to decide if new drugs have cognitive effects on the brain.

New standardized tests are always being created for neuropsychologists and older ones often need to be updated. As indicated above, in this process called standardization, "practice" versions of the new tests or tests being updated are given to many subjects so that the test developers can learn what would be considered an "average" score and what might be considered above or below average. When neuropsychologists use the final versions of these tests in their clinical settings, they then use this scaling to make decisions about their clinical patients. When tests are created, the developers also need to consider a number of other factors, such as a person's age, education level, race, ethnicity, and sex in determining the scaling for the tests. This process can take many months or years for each test, and neuropsychologists can assist at every stage of this process.

> As a clinical psychologist with a subspecialty in measurement and psychometrics, I have focused my career on creating psychological tests and measures for the clinicians who use them and outcomes scales for researchers. I have had funding from places like the National Institutes of Health (NIH), National Institute on Disability, Independent Living, and Rehabilitation Research (NIDILRR), and the Department of Defense (DOD) to create measures related to functioning and quality of life of people who have sudden and major traumatic injuries like spinal cord injury, traumatic brain injury, and limb-loss. Most important, we engage people who have a disability to identify the most important cognitive, emotional, functional, social, or physical/medical problems that disrupt their quality of life following their injuries. Once we have developed a pool of items, we "field test" these items and overall scales in large measurement studies. We utilize advanced statistical techniques that can help us evaluate how the items function as part of a scale, remove items that do not seem to measure the construct well, and then we validate the resulting measures to determine if the scale measures the constructs that we hope to assess. Finally, we have used computer technology to assist in tailoring the administration of these scales so that individuals will only receive the items that are the most discriminating for their level of functioning. I have worked in universities and medical centers and at a commercial test publishing/development company where I led the development of some of the leading tests of cognitive functioning (e.g., the Wechsler Intelligence Scales).
>
> David Tulsky, Ph.D.

I am a tenured associate professor and an associate chair for research in a clinical department in a large academic medical center. In my job, I wear a lot of hats and have responsibilities in three main areas – research, teaching, and service. My background in psychology, and neuropsychology in particular, gave me a very solid foundation in measurement. While training in measurements is an important part of psychology, it's not for most other disciplines so I am often the expert in the room. I do a lot of grant writing to attain money to develop measures, which can be a very solitary but also creative activity. When my measurement projects are funded, I lead a team of different professionals to identify what kinds of things are most important to measure within patients presenting with a certain problem, and then we develop and refine the items on the measure often through focus groups and advanced statistics. This work involves a lot of collaboration with other faculty with expertise that's very different from mine, mentorship of junior staff, and writing manuscripts about the measures so that the clinical community will know that they are available and how they were developed. I've also served on my IRB and on committees and in leadership roles in national organizations that are an important part of supporting the next generation of scientists. All in all, every day is different, and I love what I do.

Claire Kalpakjian, Ph.D., M.S.

Neuropsychologists who work for pharmaceutical companies can help to decide whether a drug that is designed to improve cognition, such as for Alzheimer's disease, is actually working. They can also help to decide whether there might be side effects of drugs designed to treat other medical or psychiatric diagnoses that may worsen a person's cognition. When pharmaceutical companies test new drugs, they enroll many people into a clinical trial. All the people in the trial are first evaluated to make sure they have the correct diagnosis that the drug is designed to treat, and there are strict guidelines about how long the people will take the drug and what their dose will be. A neuropsychologist may conduct an evaluation at the beginning of the trial, at the end of the trial, and sometimes several weeks or months after the trial is finished to see if the drug changed the person's cognition.

> While I was still a Neuropsychology graduate student, I became interested in pursuing research that could translate into new treatments for disorders of the nervous system. To be close to the translational process, I chose a research career in the biotechnology industry. In my position, I lead a team that conducts research about potential new treatments for serious disorders of the nervous system. My training in Neuropsychology provided me with a strong appreciation of the power of behavior as an elegant measure of nervous system function, and my team uses behavioral analyses extensively in our research. In addition, as potential treatments have moved from research into clinical trials, I have felt comfortable offering suggestions about potential human functional endpoints and test batteries.

Susan D. Croll, Ph.D.

Policy and Administration

In addition to or instead of any of the clinical or research roles described above, some neuropsychologists have leadership roles that allow them to help develop the specialty of neuropsychology as a whole. They may, for instance, work with licensing boards and help to set the requirements for getting licensed in a certain state. Even more commonly, they assist large organizations such as AACN or APA, or more local psychological organizations, on various committees that focus on advocacy such as: state laws and regulations related to the practice of neuropsychology, issues related to insurance, educating the public about the specialty of neuropsychology, and mentoring students of neuropsychology (especially those who live in more rural areas and may not have direct contact with licensed neuropsychologists locally). By working with larger organizations, neuropsychologists can be more coordinated in these kinds of efforts and have a stronger action plan to address these areas together. Below is a quote from a Past President of the National Academy of Neuropsychology:

> I have made professional service an integral part of my practice as a neuropsychologist and incorporated it into negotiations for my time at work. I spend at least several hours a week engaged in professional service activities (e.g., meetings, working on projects, consulting with others), which enriches my other work in many tangible and intangible ways. At least several days per year, I spend the full day involved in activities solely related to professional service, including conferences and legislative advocacy initiatives. It's great to be "in the know" about big changes in the field (e.g., changes in practice governed by the Centers for Medicare and Medicaid Services, updates to training guidelines via the Minnesota Update Conference), and I have made connections with other neuropsychologists throughout the world, gaining relationships and knowledge I would have missed if I stayed focused solely on my individual practice. I have the privilege of being involved in neuropsychology at a leadership level, and I try to consider all activities with an eye toward expanding our table for others who may not share this privilege.
>
> Beth C. Arredondo, Ph.D., ABPP-CN

Multiple Roles (Some Additional Examples by Your Authors)

Now that you know more about some settings where neuropsychologists can work and what their day-to-day activities are like in each setting, we thought we'd share a little about our roles.

One of the authors (LAS) has both a full-time job and a (at least one) part-time job, which is not all that uncommon as mentioned previously. Her full-time job is at an academic medical center, where she has multiple roles as Director of Neuropsychology Services and Training. She sees adult and older adult patients, both inpatient and outpatient, for either cognitive screens and bedside counseling (inpatient) or more comprehensive neuropsychological evaluations and psychotherapy or cognitive remediation (outpatient). She also co-leads an outpatient cognitive skills group. The patients she sees tend to either have dementia, have suffered a brain injury or stroke, or have had some other neurological illness or injury. However, she occasionally consults to the inpatient psychiatric unit as well. Dr. Schaefer supervises numerous psychology externs (graduate students) and interns, and teaches didactic seminars to both them and medical residents. Regarding research, she has presented interesting cases and also analyzed and presented data on topics such as verbal fluency in dementia and brain injury patients, and how cognition affects discharge destination in older adult stroke inpatients. Dr. Schaefer has also served on, and served as Chair of, the institutional review board (IRB) at her hospital, which reviews and approves research from various departments. Each day of the week is different, and this variety – of clinical work, teaching, research, and administration – is one of the things she loves about her job.

Her part-time job is in private practice, where she can be selective about the patients she sees. Since she only works at her private practice one night a week and the occasional weekend, she sees 2–4 patients a week for psychotherapy and occasionally an evaluation. The therapy patients all have either suffered a brain injury, stroke, or have been diagnosed with early dementia. Sometimes she also engages in forensic neuropsychology work, including IMEs, expert witness testimony, or guardianship evaluations which she conducts for the court or for attorneys. These typically require taking time off from her full-time job, though, as they can be time-consuming. Dr. Schaefer also does "per diem" (meaning "by the day") work for another hospital, on the occasional weekend; this began as coverage for another neuropsychologist when they were out on leave. Neuropsychologists are relatively scarce and in demand, so sometimes hospitals will seek someone who can cover when they have too many referrals or when their neuropsychologist is unavailable. Besides all of the above, Dr. Schaefer has written this and another book, presented at conferences, and is involved in a number of committees in neuropsychological organizations. As you can see, neuropsychologists can and do work in multiple settings and assume various roles. This variety and flexibility are strengths of the specialty, and – although sometimes tiring (see Chapter 6) – are reasons we love neuropsychology and sharing it with others.

The other author (HB) currently works in an outpatient specialty program within an academic medical center for young people experiencing an early episode of psychosis. For many years she worked at another academic medical center in an outpatient program for individuals of all ages with a variety of neurological diagnoses including traumatic brain injury, stroke, brain tumors, Parkinson's disease, and multiple sclerosis. In both settings, she has been part of interdisciplinary teams offering services such as medication management, neuropsychology, cognitive remediation, individual psychotherapy, and various forms of group therapy. When working more specifically with patients who had neurological diagnoses, there were also often speech and language pathologists, physical therapists, and occupational therapists on the treatment teams. In both settings, some of her patients have had legal cases, either civil or criminal, requiring her to interact with the legal system. Dr. Bertisch has also been very engaged in training activities; she has worked with psychology students at all levels and was the Associate Director of the Psychology Postdoctoral fellowship in her former position. In her current position she supervises medical residents as well. In addition, Dr. Bertisch has been very involved in conducting research; she regularly gives presentations, publishes papers, and has written and been funded through many research grants. As part of her research work, she trains and supervises junior research staff too. Finally, Dr. Bertisch is active in many national and local organizations which represent psychologists and neuropsychologists in the hopes of making the specialty even better on the whole.

This chapter attempted to provide the experience of "being in the shoes" of neuropsychologists in multiple (although not all possible) settings. One of the advantages of neuropsychology as a career is that a neuropsychologist can work in one of a variety of different settings, or even in multiple settings. This flexibility is wonderful especially for those of us with too many interests in the subject matter of brain and behavior, or who can't settle on or feel they might get bored with just one setting, patient population, or activity. You can still be an expert, or specialist, in neuropsychology, but do many different things and take on varying roles – either serially or simultaneously. Then again, for those who do know what they love, you can also super-specialize, focusing on one setting and diving into a particular area. It's up to you. During your training is the ideal opportunity to try and sample many different settings and populations, so that you can get a feel for what you do and do not like, and in what you may like to specialize.

References

American Board of Professional Psychology (2023). *Forensic psychology.* https://abpp.org/Applicant-Information/Specialty-Boards/Forensic-Psychology.aspx

American Psychological Association (2019, October). *Questions? We have answers: Membership in APA gives you access to consultation services from staff experts on issues impacting your work.* APA Services, Inc. https://www.apaservices.org/practice/legal/questions

Bellone, J. A., & Van Patten, R. (2021). *Becoming a neuropsychologist: Advice and guidance for students and trainees.* Springer.

Craig, P. (2017) Neuropsychologists. In Sternberg, R. J. *Career paths in psychology: Where your degree can take you.* American Psychological Association.

Custom Continuing Education, L.L.C. (n.d.). *CE requirements by state.* AllPsych. https://allpsych.com/state-ce-requirements/

Grote, C. L., Butts, A. M., & Bodin, D. (2016). Education, training and practice of clinical neuropsychologists in the United States of America. *The Clinical Neuropsychologist, 30*(8), 1356–1370.

Harvey, P. D. (2022). Clinical applications of neuropsychological assessment. *Dialogues in clinical neuroscience, 14*(1), 91–99.

Kirsch-Darrow, L., & Tsao, J. W. (2021). Cognitive rehabilitation. *CONTINUUM: Lifelong Learning in Neurology, 27*(6), 1670–1681.

Klonoff, P. S. (2010). *Psychotherapy after brain injury: Principles and techniques.* Guilford Press.

Morrison, C. E., MacAllister, W. S., & Barr, W. B. (2018). Neuropsychology within a tertiary care epilepsy center. *Archives of Clinical Neuropsychology, 33*(3), 354–364.

Parente, R., & Stapelton, M. (1997). History and systems of cognitive rehabilitation. *Neurorehabilitation*, 8, 3–11. doi: 10.3233/NRE-1997–8102.

Pepping, M. (2015). *Successful practice in neuropsychology and neuro-rehabilitation: A scientist-practitioner model.* Second Edition. Elsevier.

Postal, K. S., & Armstrong, K. (2013). *Feedback that sticks: The art of effectively communicating neuropsychological assessment results.* Oxford University Press.

Prigatano, G. P. (2005). A history of cognitive rehabilitation. In P. W. Halligan & D. T. Wade (Eds.), *The effectiveness of rehabilitation for cognitive deficits.* Oxford Scholarship Online. doi: 10.1093/acprof:oso/9780198526544.001.0001

Ruff, R. M., & Chester, S. K. (2014). *Effective psychotherapy for individuals with brain injury.* Guilford Publications.

Schaefer, L.A., & Farrer, T. J. (2022). *A casebook of mental capacity in US legislation assessment and legal commentary.* Routledge.

Sohlberg, M. M., & Mateer, C. A. (2001). *Cognitive rehabilitation: An integrative neuropsychological approach.* Guilford Press.

Sweet, J. J., Klipfel, K. M., Nelson, N. W., & Moberg, P. J. (2021). Professional practices, beliefs, and incomes of U.S. neuropsychologists: The AACN, NAN, SCN 2020 practice and "salary survey." *The Clinical Neuropsychologist, 35*, 7–80, doi: 10.1080/13854046.2020.1849803

van Heugten, C., Caldenhove, S., Crutsen, J., & Winkens, I. (2020). An overview of outcome measures used in neuropsychological rehabilitation research on adults with acquired brain injury. *Neuropsychological rehabilitation, 30*(8), 1598–1623.

4 What Kinds of Patients Do Neuropsychologists See?

Just like many other kinds of psychologists, neuropsychologists can work with people with a variety of diagnoses, ages, and cultural and family backgrounds. The commonality is that all neuropsychologists work with people who have had a problem that affected their brain, either directly or indirectly. Some neuropsychologists become interested in this subject because they want to work with a particular diagnosis or medical condition; some become interested because they like a specific age group; and others are interested in working within a particular community where certain diagnoses may more commonly be seen. Referrals tend to come from physicians (neurologists, psychiatrists, internists, physiatrists, pediatricians, and geriatricians), but can also come from other psychologists or other professionals, including attorneys (forensic issues will not be covered here, but are discussed in Chapter 3).

There are many ways to organize information about the kinds of patients that neuropsychologists tend to see, and one easy way to do so is by age group, which is how this chapter is written (Poole & Snarey, 2011). Although providing detail about each of the kinds of diagnoses outlined here is beyond the scope of this chapter, you can check The National Library of Medicine's MedlinePlus website for easy-to-read online summaries of neurologic diseases, mental disorders, and developmental disabilities (National Library of Medicine, n.d.). See also the eResources accompanying this book. It is important to recognize that in practice, real patients can actually present with multiple problems, including problems with substance abuse, other medical or psychiatric issues, family problems, and/or financial constraints that need to be considered when working with each individual case, in addition to the primary diagnosis for which the person is coming to see a neuropsychologist. In addition, although the specifics are sometimes different, some diagnoses may be seen in more than one age group, as indicated below. Some neuropsychologists focus on one age group or set of conditions, and others are considered to be "lifespan" experts and are experienced in testing people of all ages and diagnoses (Bellone & Van Patten, 2021).

DOI: 10.4324/9781003315513-4

Pediatric (Ages Infancy–18)

This age group ranges from infancy (defined as birth to 18 months) through adolescence (18 years; Poole & Snarey, 2011). Some **pediatric** neuropsychologists may practice across this age range, and others may focus on specific ages and/or developmental stages within pediatrics. Although people change tremendously as they grow from infancy to age 18, common reasons any in this age group come to see a neuropsychologist include: 1) developmental reasons, 2) academic or school-related reasons, 3) medical reasons, and 4) psychiatric reasons. Each of these reasons can cause problems with a child or adolescent's thinking skills, and the **pediatric neuropsychologist** can use the results of their standardized assessment to get help for the child in school or in other places where the child spends time. Sometimes the child might have more than one of these problems or conditions.

Developmental Disabilities

According to the Centers for Disease Control and Prevention (CDC), "developmental disabilities are a group of conditions due to an impairment in physical, learning, language, or behavior areas. These conditions begin during the developmental period, may impact day-to-day functioning, and usually last throughout a person's lifetime" (Centers for Disease Control and Prevention, 2022a). Examples of developmental disabilities include Down syndrome, autism spectrum disorders, fetal alcohol syndrome, birth trauma, and sometimes prematurity. Pediatric neuropsychologists can use special standardized tests even for young infants to better understand how a known developmental disability may be impacting a child's **sensorimotor skills** and ability to perceive the world, explore the world, think about the world, remember, and communicate (Johnson et al., 2014). The results can then be used to help make recommendations for **early intervention**, which allows the child to receive services like speech therapy, occupational therapy, or physical therapy even before starting school to help them improve in the areas where they are delayed (Centers for Disease Control and Prevention, 2022b).

Learning Disabilities and ADHD

Many children experience difficulties learning in school, or academic problems, for a variety of reasons. Sometimes this can be related to known developmental delays, but a child can also have other problems with learning, which usually aren't noticed until the child starts school. For instance, a learning disability can cause a child to reverse letters, words, or numbers, or to have problems understanding or remembering instructions or other information. Problems with these skills can then cause the child to have difficulty in subjects like math or reading in school. A child may also have problems with focusing and/or impulsivity that results in a diagnosis of attention-deficit/hyperactivity disorder (ADHD). A pediatric neuropsychologist can use their tests to better understand these kinds of problems. They will then share the results of the evaluation with the child's school, which typically includes the school psychologist. The neuropsychologist will work with the school to come up with a plan to teach the child differently and/or help them in the areas where they have difficulty. These plans are often designed as Individualized Educational Plans (IEP) or Section 504 plans (deBettencourt, 2002). Sometimes the neuropsychologist will also re-evaluate the child over time to measure their progress.

Medical

Although it is less common in this age group, people who were born healthy can sometimes suffer from serious medical conditions later in childhood or adolescence, such as cancer, strokes, traumatic brain injuries, multiple sclerosis, epilepsy, or infections that can affect the brain and cognition. For these individuals, a pediatric neuropsychologist can use children's versions of various standardized tests to measure the child's ability to focus, remember, organize, and **problem-solve** in order to understand how their problems in these areas can affect schoolwork and their ability to make and keep friends. The neuropsychologist would then share this information with the child's school and, similarly to how it is done for a child with a learning disability, the school and the neuropsychologist would work together to develop a plan, possibly an IEP or a Section 504 plan, to help the child succeed in classes and/or socially.

Psychiatric Disorders and Addiction

Finally, although it is more often recognized in adolescents, some people are surprised to learn that younger children can also experience significant mental health problems that may impact their cognition. These include anxiety, depression, obsessive compulsive disorder (OCD), post-traumatic stress disorder (PTSD), and even psychosis (Merikangas et al., 2009). They may also exhibit behavioral disturbances where they have difficulty following rules and controlling their anger. Especially in adolescence, they may start using alcohol or drugs so much that it interferes with their schoolwork, relationships with family and friends, or their safety. Sometimes these problems happen in combination with other developmental, learning, or medical issues. For these children and adolescents, a referral to a pediatric neuropsychologist who can utilize tests to better understand any cognitive or behavioral problems can help with creating an academic plan with the school as described above. Assessment results can also be used by a mental health treatment team to understand how the child or adolescent's cognitive and behavioral problems can be helped by the services they are providing, and how to manage them.

Case Examples

Early Childhood Traumatic Brain Injury.

An 8-year-old male suffered a traumatic brain injury, including frontal sub-dural hematoma, after being hit by a car while riding his bicycle. He spent four weeks in the hospital, and another four weeks being home-schooled. He complained of headache and memory problems. His pediatrician and school requested neuropsychological testing to assess his cognitive functioning. Dr. Jones, a pediatric neuropsychologist, performed the evaluation, which showed problems with attention, distractibility, encoding, processing speed, and inhibition, as well as some depression. Dr. Jones reported this to the elementary school and to the pediatrician, and recommended counseling as well as academic accommodations when he returned to school. The testing also served as a baseline, to compare to later testing to document improvement.

First Episode Psychosis.

A 16-year-old male patient was recently discharged from an inpatient psychiatric hospitalization. His symptoms were hearing voices and expressing unusual beliefs and behaviors, and he was given a diagnosis of schizophreniform disorder. Prior to his hospitalization, his grades also began to decline and he said that he was having trouble focusing and organizing his schoolwork. Dr. Lee, a neuropsychologist, gave him neuropsychological tests and found that his performance in the areas of speed, attention, memory, organization, and problem-solving were lower than would be expected. Dr. Lee was then able to share this information with both his mental health treatment team and his high school and they were able to develop a plan, including cognitive remediation, to help him.

Young and Middle Adulthood (Ages 19–64)

Medical

Although some medical problems are more commonly seen in younger adulthood, for instance multiple sclerosis, the risk of many medical problems increases as a person gets older. Below is a list of medical problems that can affect the brain for which adults would generally see a neuropsychologist:

- Traumatic brain injury
- Multiple sclerosis
- Stroke
- Aneurysm

- Loss of oxygen to the brain (sometimes due to heart problems or drug overdose)
- Brain infections or inflammation
- Parkinson's disease and related diseases
- Seizure disorders
- Cancer (i.e., brain tumors or the impact of treatment for other cancers on the brain)
- Non-cancerous brain tumors or cysts

Psychiatric Disorders and Addiction

Many serious psychiatric disorders are diagnosed in late adolescence or early adulthood. These include depression, bipolar disorder, OCD, PTSD, and psychotic disorders like schizophrenia. Because all of these conditions are brain-related, they can also affect a person's cognition. In addition, when people have problems with substance abuse, involving either alcohol or other drugs, these substances can also affect the brain and thinking skills, especially if they are taken in large doses and/or over time. Often, people with serious mental health diagnoses also abuse drugs or alcohol. A neuropsychologist who works in this area will understand how the mental health condition and/or problem with substance abuse can affect the brain. They can use standardized tests to better understand the resulting cognitive problems for a particular individual, and then work with that individual's therapist, family, or other caretakers to come up with a plan for how these difficulties can be managed.

Early Onset Dementias and Mild Cognitive Impairment (MCI)

Most of the time, people who develop dementias such as Alzheimer's disease are diagnosed later in life, and these conditions are therefore described in the section on older adults below. The diagnosis may be contingent on a number of **risk factors** a person has, however, and some dementias, including frontotemporal dementia, are typically diagnosed when a person is a bit younger. When assessing dementias, a neuropsychologist will often conduct follow-up evaluations to monitor how the illness is progressing.

In addition, some people may come to a neuropsychologist with a condition called mild cognitive impairment (MCI; Palmer et al., 2003). With MCI, a person may be showing signs of problems with memory or language more than other people their age, but is still able to take care of themselves and manage their life overall. Some people with MCI will go on to develop dementia, some people will not, and some people will improve, depending on what is causing the problem. Therefore, it is important for the neuropsychologist and others working with this person to monitor their cognition over time to decide if they will need additional care.

Case Examples

Adult Traumatic Brain Injury.

A 51-year-old female hit her head during a car accident. She was in the hospital for a week and tried to go back to her job as a lawyer afterwards. She had a lot of trouble remembering appointments and deadlines, which caused problems for her law firm. Dr. Smith, a neuropsychologist, gave her a neuropsychological evaluation and discovered that she was struggling with focus, memory, and organization compared to what she was likely able to do before her accident. Dr. Smith recommended cognitive remediation and helped her to work out a plan with her job to have fewer responsibilities initially, tapering up as she continued to heal.

Long-COVID.

A 33-year-old male suffered from a severe bought of COVID-19 in late spring of 2020. He had acute symptoms for two months, and was bedridden for four months, suffering from extreme fatigue, decreased oxygen saturation, difficulty with memory recall, and inability to speak at times. He had been a graduate student at this time and had to drop out the spring semester and took a leave for the fall semester. When he returned, he needed extra time and a reduced course load. One year after his acute illness, his neurologist referred him for testing. The neuropsychologist, Dr. Garcia, administered a comprehensive battery of tests to delineate the patient's strengths and weaknesses. Although his memory had improved, the patient still had difficulties with attention and learning, as well as with multi-tasking. Dr. Garcia recommended cognitive remediation and continued to work with his graduate school for accommodations.

Older Adulthood (Ages 65 and Older)

Medical

As it was noted above, the risk of many medical conditions increases as a person ages. This is in part related to family history, the presence of other medical conditions such as diabetes or high blood pressure and how well these conditions are managed, and how well a person takes care of themselves overall. The medical conditions listed in the "Young and Middle Adulthood" section above may therefore be even more commonly seen in older adults. Older adults are a group that is also at greater risk for traumatic brain injury due to falls (Harvey and Close, 2012).

Psychiatric Disorders and Addiction

All of the psychiatric disorders noted above can also be seen in older adults. Depending on the setting and why the person is coming to see a neuropsychologist, they may have had a long history of mental illness (i.e., schizophrenia or PTSD), or it may be a newer problem, such as depression. Older adults actually have lower rates of depression than younger adults, but higher rates of completed suicide. Depression may be caused by having more stress such as caring for a sick loved one or managing their own illnesses, financial stresses, or because of loneliness and isolation that happens more often in this age group (Kok and Reynolds, 2017). In older adults, depression can also look similar to dementia, and it is important for the neuropsychologist to use their standardized tests to distinguish between the two conditions to help the client get the appropriate treatment (Kok and Reynolds, 2017).

Although it is most prevalent in young adulthood, some people are surprised to learn that substance abuse is also common in older adulthood (Kuerbis et al., 2014). This includes alcohol, illicit substances, and misuse of prescription medications. Sometimes the impact of substance abuse can be confused with symptoms of other chronic illnesses, especially in older adults, and it is important that the neuropsychologist determines what is really causing the symptoms to help the client get the correct treatment. As older adults metabolize substances differently, it is especially important that substance abuse and the reasons why the person is abusing the substance are treated appropriately in this age group.

Dementia

As the brain ages, dementia becomes more common. Dementia is actually not just one thing, but an overall term used to describe a set of **progressive** or gradually worsening conditions that can impact a person's: memory, language, other cognitive skills, ability to care for themselves, ability to work, ability to enjoy the things they used to, and ability to keep up with friends and family (Arvanitakis and Bennett, 2019). The most common form of dementia is Alzheimer's disease, but there are others, including vascular dementia and Lewy Body dementia. Neuropsychologists utilize testing in combination with their knowledge of each of the kinds of dementia to decide whether their client has dementia and, if so, what type they have. This is important in deciding what to expect in terms of how the dementia will progress, what kind of care might be needed, and whether the client will likely respond to the treatments that are available. Although there is no "cure" for most dementias at this time, there are treatments that can help improve a person's cognition and functioning for as long as possible with some kinds of dementia. The neuropsychologist will most likely do follow-up evaluations with a person who has dementia to monitor how their illness is progressing and update decisions about their care based on this information.

End-of-Life Care

There are several reasons a neuropsychologist may be involved in a person's end-of-life care at any age. One, as described earlier in this section and in the section on nursing homes in Chapter 3, it is important to understand where a person may be in the course of a chronic or progressive illness in order to decide what kind or amount of care may be best. Also, neuropsychological evaluation or consultation can be helpful in determining whether a person is able to think clearly enough to make decisions about their own care, or whether they will need help with decision-making going forward (Kolva et al., 2020; Schaefer & Farrer, 2022).

Case Example

Dementia.

An 82-year-old female was brought in for testing by her daughter. According to the daughter, the patient had a lot of trouble over the past two years remembering conversations, forgetting to take her medication, and losing things in her home. Dr. Brown, a neuropsychologist, reviewed the patient's medical records, interviewed both the patient and her daughter, and administered a neuropsychological assessment. Dr. Brown discovered that her delayed memory, naming, ability to shift ideas, and abstract reasoning were well below that of other people her age. After ruling out treatable causes, Dr. Brown felt that the patient had Alzheimer's disease. They scheduled a feedback session to go over the results with the patient and her family, and made a number of recommendations, including cognitive strategies, referral to a neurologist for possible medication, and supervision at home for her safety.

In conclusion, neuropsychologists work with patients from infancy to end-of-life, with developmental problems, brain injuries, medical/neurological or psychiatric illnesses, and/or addictions. Some choose to specialize in a particular age group or disorder, while others see patients throughout the lifespan and work with multiple conditions. It is this variety and flexibility that makes the specialty so interesting and provides multiple opportunities to the future neuropsychologist.

References

Arvanitakis, Z., & Bennett, D. A. (2019). What is dementia? *Journal of the American Medical Association (JAMA), 322*(17), 1728–1728.

Bellone, J. A., & Van Patten, R. (2021). *Becoming a neuropsychologist: Advice and guidance for students and trainees).* Springer.

Centers for Disease Control and Prevention (2022a, April 27). *Facts about Developmental Disabilities.* U.S. Department of Health and Human Services. https://www.cdc.gov/ncbddd/developmentaldisabilities/facts.html

Centers for Disease Control and Prevention (2022b, August 9). *What is "Early Intervention?"* U.S. Department of Health and Human Services. https://www.cdc.gov/ncbddd/actearly/parents/states.html

deBettencourt, L. U. (2002). Understanding the differences between IDEA and Section 504. *Teaching Exceptional Children, 34*(3), 16–23.

Harvey, L. A., & Close, J. C. (2012). Traumatic brain injury in older adults: Characteristics, causes and consequences. *Injury, 43*(11), 1821–1826.

Johnson S., Moore T., & Marlow, N. (2014). Using the Bayley-III to assess neurodevelopmental delay: Which cut-off should be used? *Pediatric Research, 75,* 670–674. doi: 10.1038/pr.2014.10.

Kok, R. M., & Reynolds, C. F. (2017). Management of depression in older adults: A review. *Journal of the American Medical Association (JAMA), 317*(20), 2114–2122.

Kolva, E., Rosenfeld, B. & Saracino, R. M. (2020). Neuropsychological predictors of decision-making capacity in terminally ill patients with advanced cancer. *Archives of Clinical Neuropsychology, 35,* 1–9. doi: 10.1093/arclin/acz027

Kuerbis, A., Sacco, P., Blazer, D. G., & Moore, A. A. (2014). Substance abuse among older adults. *Clinics in Geriatric Medicine, 30*(3), 629–654.

Merikangas, K. R., Nakamura, E. F., & Kessler, R. C. (2009). Epidemiology of mental disorders in children and adolescents. *Dialogues in Clinical Neuroscience, 11*(1): 7–20. doi: 10.31887/DCNS.2009.11.1/krmerikangas

National Library of Medicine (n.d.). *Medline Plus.* National Institute of Health, U.S. Department of Health and Human Services. Retrieved January 29, 2023, from https://medlineplus.gov

Palmer, K., Fratiglioni, L., & Winblad, B. (2003). What is mild cognitive impairment? Variations in definitions and evolution of nondemented persons with cognitive impairment. *Acta Neurologica Scandinavica, 107,* 14–20.

Poole S., & Snarey J. (2011). Erikson's stages of the life cycle. In Goldstein, S., & Naglieri, J.A. (Eds.) *Encyclopedia of child behavior and development.* Springer. doi: 10.1007/978-0-387-79061-9_1024

Schaefer, L.A., & Farrer, T. J. (2022). *A casebook of mental capacity in US legislation assessment and legal commentary.* Routledge.

5 How to Become a Neuropsychologist

Three Typical Paths

Chapter 1 describes some of the interests that lead people towards the specialty of neuropsychology. With these interests as a start, there are currently three possible routes a person can take to become a neuropsychologist once they have completed their undergraduate coursework. Of note, the descriptions below are specific to the U.S. and countries with similar training to the U.S.; please refer to local requirements and regulations for other countries. See Hokkanen et al. (2020) for more on the development of neuropsychology in Europe, and Ponsford (2017) for non-Western countries and continents. In the U.S., it can take five to seven years and sometimes more to finish doctoral training in psychology, so it is important that students have both passion for their work and sufficient financial resources to be able to complete the process, which should be thought through in advance. For most psychology doctoral programs in general, there are certain undergraduate prerequisite courses that can vary a bit by the specific program. A Bachelor's degree in psychology is usually enough to cover these requirements.

A Doctoral Degree in Clinical Psychology, with a Focus on Neuropsychology

The vast majority of people who become neuropsychologists begin with a doctoral degree in clinical psychology. According to one survey, approximately 82% of all neuropsychologists have a doctoral degree in clinical psychology and 6% have a degree in counseling psychology (Sweet et al., 2021). When somebody who would like to become a neuropsychologist is selecting a clinical psychology program for their doctoral degree, it is important that they consider whether that program will: 1) offer coursework in neuropsychology, 2) have at least one option for a mentor who is a neuropsychologist and can help with decisions about where to train and how to write a dissertation relevant to the specialty, and 3) offer opportunities for hands-on training in neuropsychology. Although the degree will be in clinical (or counseling)

DOI: 10.4324/9781003315513-5

psychology, if the majority of the experiences that the student selects are relevant to neuropsychology then they will be positioned very well for a career in this specialty. Ideally, the doctoral program will be **accredited**, or recognized, by the American Psychological Association (APA) for meeting certain standards. It is highly recommended that the student chooses an APA-accredited program, as this will affect career decisions, including board certification, later (see below).

A Specialized Track, Major, or Concentration in Neuropsychology

There are no longer doctoral programs in clinical neuropsychology; ones that previously existed have been restructured into clinical psychology programs (in order to become APA accredited; APA does not accredit neuropsychology programs). There are, however, several clinical psychology programs in the United States and Canada that offer a formal track, major/minor, specialty, or concentration specifically in neuropsychology (Perry & Boccaccini, 2009). The student therefore has less to consider when deciding on such a program, as all courses, **mentorship**, and training experiences are already geared towards the subject. The student should still make sure that there are opportunities offered that are relevant to their specific interests within the specialty of neuropsychology (i.e., which patient populations they would most like to work with), however. Given that there are fewer of these programs, it is also important to think about whether the cost and/or the possibility of moving to another place to attend school is realistic for an extended period of time.

A Re-Specialization in Neuropsychology

Sometimes somebody has already received graduate-level training in another area of psychology, but would later like to change their career path to neuropsychology. The good news is that it is possible to change, or **"re-specialize"** in neuropsychology, after you have already received graduate training in another area of psychology, and even after you have completed your doctoral degree. You can even re-specialize from a non-psychology field. The amount of additional training you would need to re-specialize, of course, depends mainly on how much (if any) training you have already had in neuropsychology or a closely related field.

If the doctoral degree was already in a clinical area of psychology (i.e., clinical psychology, but without any neuropsychology training), then one would likely need at least a postdoctoral fellowship in neuropsychology in order to become a neuropsychologist, to attain that specialty training. If their doctorate was in a non-clinical field of psychology (i.e., cognitive psychology; developmental psychology), however, then one would first need to take coursework to re-specialize, and then would need to complete clinical externships, an internship, and a postdoctoral fellowship. One example of such a re-specialization program is through Fielding Graduate University. They would not need to complete a new dissertation. Lastly, if one is coming from another mental health occupation altogether (i.e., social work), or any other non-psychology field, they would have to apply to graduate doctoral programs in clinical psychology. If they did not major in psychology at the undergraduate level, they would first have to take post-baccalaureate courses to fulfill any pre-requisites before they applied. Bellone & Van Patten (2021) provide an overview of re-specialization and some additional common scenarios.

What Is Doctoral Training in Psychology Like?

Although each clinical psychology doctoral program is designed somewhat differently and each may have a different emphasis on clinical work versus research and/or a different clinical orientation (i.e., cognitive behavioral versus psychodynamic versus **eclectic**, or integrated, approaches), the general format across doctoral programs is similar. This section is designed to provide a brief overview of what the doctoral requirements and time frames are like. We suggest you also read the chapter called "Doctoral Training" in Bellone & Van Patten (2021) for additional information on this topic, as well as view websites corresponding to this chapter on the eResources included with this volume. Basically, neuropsychology training follows what is known as the Houston Conference guidelines (Hannay et al., 1998), which delineated a model for acceptable and expected education and training for the specialty of clinical neuropsychology. These are currently being updated via the Minnesota Conference (see Chapter 7 for more details).

All psychology doctoral programs require students to successfully complete coursework, usually during the first three or four years of the program. For somebody who is aspiring to become a neuropsychologist, it is important to select a program that offers coursework in neuropsychology. Relevant coursework would include neuropsychological assessment, but can also include neuroanatomy, neurophysiology, psychopharmacology, or other neuroscience or cognitive courses. During the first three or four years, students will also be required to complete several externships, or part-time and usually unpaid clinical training experiences, at any number of nearby hospitals or clinics that typically have a relationship with their doctoral program (Bornstein, 1988; Nelson et al., 2015). It would be relevant for the student to select externships that have a component of hands-on training in neuropsychological assessment and, if possible, cognitive remediation (described in Chapter 3). During these years students will also be participating to various extents in research activities, typically through a professor's lab with the same interests. This research will lead to the dissertation project, which is usually the final requirement to earn the doctoral degree. Towards the end of the doctoral training (commonly in the fifth or sixth year), students also complete a year of full-time (and typically paid) internship training at a clinic or hospital. Most doctoral programs are affiliated with a national internship consortium where students may select, interview, and match with internship sites around the country. In order to become a neuropsychologist, it is important to select an internship program with training experience in neuropsychology-related activities (Kellogg et al., 2021). One should again seek to attain an internship which is APA accredited.

Training is not complete once you receive your doctoral degree. In order to become a licensed psychologist, you need to attain additional hours of experience after you receive your degree. The number of hours and the types of activities that "count" towards these hours vary by state, but they always need to be supervised by a psychologist who is already licensed. Many people earn these hours in the form of a formal postdoctoral fellowship program (Bodin, 2021; Bornstein, 1988), which can require another application process. In fact, according to the Houston Conference, a clinical neuropsychologist is required to have had the equivalent of two full-time years of experience and specialized training, at least one of which is at the postdoctoral (residency) level (Hannay et al., 1998).

In order to eventually earn Board Certification in Clinical Neuropsychology, which is currently strongly encouraged but not required, a student needs to earn *two* years of supervised experience in the specialty of neuropsychology after they earn the doctoral degree. This is often attained via a postdoctoral fellowship. Board Certification is the final step in becoming a neuropsychologist (Grote et al., 2021); it involves peer review to determine that you are competent in the specialty. There are currently two national organizations that oversee this process and issue the certificates: The American Board of Clinical Neuropsychology (ABCN), through the American Board of Professional Psychology (ABPP), and the American Board of Professional Neuropsychology (ABN). To earn the certificate, each requires: 1) a review and approval of the applicant's experience by the board, 2) passing a written test, 3) acceptance of case write-ups, and 4) passing an oral examination. It should be noted that, as of 2018, the ABPP requires doctoral degrees to be accredited by the APA or CPA (Canadian Psychological Association) and, as of 2020, internships also have to be accredited by the APA or CPA (American Board of Professional Psychology, 2023). Applicants have up to seven years to complete this process, although many do so in less time. Although Board Certification is the last formal step in the credentialing process to become a clinical neuropsychologist, in order to keep your license psychologists are required to continually earn Continuing Education credits throughout their careers, as noted in Chapter 3 (Cox & Grus, 2019). Board certification also requires periodic maintenance of certification (MOC; see Chapter 6). Beyond board certification, there is currently an additional Pediatric Neuropsychology sub-specialization offered by ABCN, for those specializing in pediatric cases (this sub-specialty certification is *after* the original board certification).

Ph.D. versus Psy.D.

One of the most common questions asked about applying to graduate school for psychology is the difference between the Doctor of Philosophy (Ph.D.) and Doctor of Psychology (Psy.D.) degrees. In many ways they are similar. Both offer long (i.e., a minimum of 5 years) and intensive training in advanced psychology with the end goal of earning a doctorate in psychology. Both will expose you to a range of learning experiences and people in the field who will help to shape the beginning of your career. In order to go in the direction you would like, you will also need to select programs that offer matching experiences, regardless of whether it is a Ph.D. or a Psy.D. program. If you are entering the specialty of neuropsychology through the Clinical Psychology route described above, as mentioned you should select a program where there is at least one mentor who is a neuropsychologist, and ideally who works with the kinds of patients and/or does the kind of research that you are most interested in. There should also be coursework in neuropsychology and a history of students going to training sites with a focus on neuropsychology. Whether you are in a Ph.D. or a Psy.D. program this will help you to gain both experiences and contacts in the specialty. It is helpful, although not entirely necessary, to go to school in an area where you can imagine working one day since the people you meet in graduate school can perhaps later help you get a job. With a few exceptions mentioned below, either a Ph.D. or a Psy.D. can prepare you for working as a neuropsychologist in many kinds of clinical settings depending on the training experiences that you attain in either kind of program. However, the majority (over 80%) of neuropsychologists surveyed reported having a Ph.D. (Sweet et al., 2021). There are also a very small number of neuropsychologists who are Ed.D., or Doctor of Education, by training, but because this is atypical, we won't be reviewing that path here.

Although there are some common aspects of doctoral training programs in clinical psychology that are needed to become accredited by the APA, each program is designed differently. In general, however, Ph.D. programs have more emphasis on research, so the biggest difference between Ph.D. and Psy.D. programs is that a Ph.D. can offer a stronger start towards a research or academic teaching career. In the more traditional model of a Ph.D. program, students enter the program through a mentor's lab, and working with clinical patients may be less of a focus during their training, at least initially. In other models, however, the prospective student is selected into the program as a whole, but their research lab experience is still one of the most important parts of their training. In either model, the Ph.D. research expectations are more rigorous, and students may be expected to publish one or more papers and present their research at conferences, with the support of their mentors. As a bonus, however, Ph.D. students often receive a **stipend** or a small salary to work in a lab (or teach), which can help to decrease the cost of graduate school. Although the Ph.D. may be a better fit for somebody who wants a strong career in research, it is possible to find a good research mentor within a Psy.D. program and to start to build a career in research there as well.

Whereas Psy.D. programs are usually more clinically focused, Ph.D. programs vary in terms of their balances between research and clinical work. Students often ask whether one type of program is seen as "better" than the other, but the truth is that it really depends on the reputation of the specific program and the fit between the program and the student, more so than the type of degree. If somebody is looking for a strong clinical career in a particular part of the country, for instance, then a reputable Psy.D. program that matches their clinical interests in the place where they would like to practice may be a better fit than a Ph.D. program with less of a clinical focus in another part of the country. In fact, it has been shown that "research and clinical 'fit' within the program in which [the student is] applying, as well as general interpersonal skills and intellect... emerged as important admissions factors" across Clinical and Counseling Ph.D. and Psy.D. programs (Karazsia & Smith, 2016, p. 305). Some considerations for Psy.D. programs, however, include: that the class size can be larger; the programs may be free-standing and not affiliated with a university psychology department; and, as the student may not be spending as much time working in a research lab as part of the training, there may be less opportunity to receive a stipend from the program. Overall, students from Psy.D. programs tend to graduate with more debt (Grote et al., 2016).

The Finances

Graduate training costs money. Just like getting an undergraduate degree, however, the amount depends on a large number of factors including: 1) the tuition for the school, 2) whether a stipend is offered and, if so, how much it is, 3) the cost of living in the area where the school is located, 4) whether it is possible for a student to do paid work in addition to the requirements of the program, and 5) the student's personal financial resources. Some schools (typically Ph.D., rather than Psy.D., programs) offer tuition remission plus a small stipend in exchange for teaching or research responsibilities, but not all programs do. Make sure you investigate this when looking at programs. One survey showed that about a third of neuropsychology doctoral students leave training with minimal debt, but almost half finish their degrees owing over $100,000 (Whiteside et al., 2016). It is important to remember that student loans will need to be paid back with additional interest, and expected starting salaries are generally in the $80–100,000 range (Whiteside et al., 2016). There are loan repayment programs, for instance through the National Institutes of Health, however, that can help offset these costs (National Institutes of Health, n.d.). It is hoped that there will be more such programs that are offered to students with loans in the future.

Should I Get a Master's Degree First?

In some cases, it may be helpful to get your Master's degree before moving on to a doctoral program in psychology, and in other cases it may not. This section outlines the pros and cons of getting a Master's degree before applying for a doctoral degree.

Pros

Getting a Master's degree first may be helpful if there are areas in your undergraduate experience that you would like to improve to give yourself a stronger application for doctoral programs. A Master's degree, for instance, may help to balance out a lower undergraduate GPA and show that you have become more focused on a career as a neuropsychologist over time. It can also be helpful if you would like further opportunity to add more research experience to your resume, which is always an asset for doctoral programs. Further, if your undergraduate degree is not in psychology or you didn't take the core psychology courses required for graduate school (these may vary by school, but typically include Introduction to Psychology, statistics, research methods, experimental psychology, and we highly recommend physiological psychology), you will need to first take some courses, whether or not in a formal post-baccalaureate or Master's program (see above), before applying for the doctorate.

Some people who are interested in the subject matter of neuropsychology do not wish to go on for a full doctoral degree. A Master's degree is a great option for someone who might want to become a **psychometrician**, or a person who administers neuropsychological tests and collects data for a doctoral-level neuropsychologist, or a research technician who can use the tests within the context of research studies under the supervision of a senior researcher.

Alternatively, a Master's degree in psychology can be used as a prerequisite for other psychology-related positions, such as a Licensed Mental Health Counselor in New York State (see Chapter 2 for other job descriptions and requirements).

Cons

The primary "con" of earning a Master's degree first is that it is not an endpoint to becoming a neuropsychologist who can practice independently. Master's degree programs can be costly and the amount would be in addition to the costs accrued from your doctoral program and any undergraduate loans. Sometimes credits don't directly transfer from Master's degree to doctoral programs, especially if they are at different universities. This may mean that you would still have to take a comparable number of doctoral courses to earn your degree. Even if it is the same university that you wish to apply, some programs won't take their own Master's degree (or undergraduate) students for the doctorate; you have to check with the specific program. Finally, as most programs offer Master's degrees in the course of earning your doctoral degree anyway, you will already be receiving a Master's degree along the way.

Gaining Clinically-Related and Research Experience

A strong undergraduate GPA is a starting point to a compelling application for graduate school, as is membership in honor societies such as Psi Chi, Nu Rho Psi, and/or Phi Beta Kappa. However, respectable grades and Graduate Record Examination (GRE) scores are not enough. Gaining hands-on applied experience with the kinds of patients you think you would like to work will both help you to know what it is really like to work with these individuals in actual settings, and it will show the professors reviewing your application that you are coming in to graduate school already "knowing your stuff." The clinical work that you do in graduate school will then be built upon the experiences you've already had. Many universities and hospitals offer a variety of internships, summer opportunities, and volunteer positions in a range of settings that can help you find these experiences as an undergraduate. Of course, since you are likely not yet licensed in anything, the definition of "clinical" experience is fairly broad. Even if you cannot get experience working with patients, gaining experience with particular age groups (i.e., older adults, children) can help determine your likes and dislikes as well as show admissions committees that you can work with people. Other ideas include working with people with disabilities, as a camp counselor, at a suicide hotline or text-line, as an EMT, as a hospital/psychiatric center/nursing home volunteer, or as a scribe. Tutoring or TA experiences are also beneficial. Even retail or food service work can broadly count as experience working with others, especially if you took on a leadership role; you can supplement this with another, more "clinical," experience. Unfortunately, the COVID-19 pandemic limited the number and types of experiences – both clinical and research – that may have previously been available to students. Thankfully, as of this date, availability is starting to improve again. In addition, everyone is in the same boat in this regard, and graduate schools and admissions committees are aware of the situation. Just keep in mind that it may take longer to get the requisite experiences because of this, and there will be stiffer competition.

Having research experience is especially important for a strong graduate school application. This is important even if you do not think you ultimately want to become a researcher, because to be a good clinician you will need to be able to learn from the research and understand how research studies are conducted. If you would like to pursue a career in research, undergraduate research experience will allow you to learn the "basics" so that you can more easily continue in this direction in graduate school. As noted in Chapter 3, many university professors have research labs and can often use the help of undergraduate students to keep things running smoothly. This is a perfect opportunity for you to see first-hand how research is conducted, and to be able to show this knowledge on your graduate school applications. When applying to graduate school, demonstrating research "goodness of fit" with graduate faculty's research interests and expertise may make you a more preferred candidate for that program (Karazsia et al., 2013).

While conducting research, it is optimal to see studies through to their completion as attending professional conferences, presenting posters, and assisting with publications can be particularly exciting, and look especially good on an application or CV (curriculum vitae). By working in someone's lab, you will also get to know the professor and they will get to know you. This is important when it comes to obtaining letters of recommendation. The better the professors get to know you and your work, the stronger the letter they can write. Other ways to get to know professors include serving as a teaching assistant or regularly attending office hours (in addition to class).

Chapter 1, entitled "Applying and Getting into Graduate School," in Cady Kristen Block's book *The Neuropsychologist's Roadmap: A Training and Career Guide* (2021) provides an excellent description about the kinds of experience that graduate schools look for in an application and what the application process is like (Suhr et al., 2021).

Other Advice

Even with a solid undergraduate GPA and/or a Master's degree and having had good clinical and research experience before your doctoral training, it is very common for doctoral applicants to worry that their applications aren't "good enough." Doctoral programs are extremely competitive, so this is a realistic concern. On a practical level, it is a good idea to sit down with a trusted mentor or a professor before applying to graduate school, to get an outside opinion on where you may be able to improve your profile before you apply. Sometimes this requires a gap year, to gain more experience (neither of your authors took a gap year, so we cannot comment too much here, however we might be in the minority if we were applying today). It is also important, however, to know that there is no such thing as a "perfect" application. Some people may not have scored as highly as they had hoped on their GRE, and others may feel they could have had even more clinical or research experience. Most graduate programs will review your application as a whole, and any relative weakness can be addressed in a cover letter with your application. They will likely want to invite you in for an interview if you make the first cut. If your overall application is strong, an area or two of weakness is less relevant to the "big picture." Arguably, the most important factor is the "fit" between you and the program, as we have been saying, and you will want to establish that in your personal statement, where you will discuss your interests and goals.

First Steps

A directory of specific doctoral programs in clinical psychology with training in neuropsychology is beyond the scope of this book, and frankly would be a book unto itself. One suggestion is to join the American Psychological Association (APA) as a Student Member (currently for $35/year for undergraduates) at www.apa.org which gives you 25% off all APA books and DVDs. Then you can get discounted access to the "Graduate Study in Psychology" database, of programs throughout the U.S. and Canada. You can search for programs in Clinical Psychology that have some training, or a formal track or concentration, in neuropsychology (as mentioned, some people enter neuropsychology by way of a Counseling Psychology program, but that is atypical). Some other books sold by APA include: *Getting In: A Step-by-Step Plan for Gaining Admission to Graduate School in Psychology, Second Edition* (2007) and *Applying to Graduate School in Psychology: Advice from Successful Students and Prominent Psychologists* (2008) by Kracen and Wallace. Another book suggestion is the *Insider's Guide to Graduate Programs in Clinical and Counseling Psychology* (Norcross and Sayette, 2022), which provides a guide for prospective graduate students as well as a review of individual programs. Find out what is required from different programs, as there is currently no "common application." If you are not geographically tied to an area, you increase your options and better your chances of admission if you can apply throughout the country. This may sound intimidating, but will ultimately broaden your network and you may find you love living in a different part of the country.

The process of researching programs and applying to graduate school is time-consuming and may be anxiety-producing. However, knowledge of the process and your options will serve you well during this exciting time of your life and help you to make the best decisions.

References

American Board of Professional Psychology (2023). *General requirements.* https://abpp.org/application-information/general-requirements/

American Psychological Association (2007). *Getting in: A step-by-step plan for gaining admission to graduate school in psychology, 2nd Edition.* American Psychological Association.

Bellone, J. A. & Van Patten, R. (2021). *Becoming a neuropsychologist: Advice and guidance for students and trainees.* Springer.

Bodin, D. (2021). Preparing for and obtaining a postdoctoral fellowship. In C. K. Block (Ed.) *The neuropsychologist's roadmap: A training and career guide* (pages 55–72). American Psychological Association.

Bornstein, R. A. (1988). Entry into clinical neuropsychology: Graduate, undergraduate, and beyond. *The Clinical Neuropsychologist, 2,* 213–220, doi: 10.1080/13854048808520103

Cox, D. R., & Grus, C. L. (2019). From continuing education to continuing competence. *Professional Psychology: Research and Practice, 50*(2), 113.

Grote, C. L., Butts, A. M., & Bodin, D. (2016). Education, training and practice of clinical neuropsychologists in the United States of America. *The Clinical Neuropsychologist, 30*(8), 1356–1370.

Grote, C., Soble, J., R., & León, A. (2021). Board certification in neuropsychology. In C. K. Block (Ed.) *The neuropsychologist's roadmap: A training and career guide* (pages 89–108). American Psychological Association.

Hannay, H. J., Bieliauskas, L., Crosson, B. A., Hammeke, T. A., Hamsher, K. D., & Koffler, S. (1998). Proceedings of the Houston Conference on Specialty Education and Training in Clinical Neuropsychology. *Archives of Clinical Neuropsychology, 13*(2), 157–250.

Hokkanen, L., Barbosa, F., Ponchel, A., Constantinou, M., Kosmidis, M. H., Varako, N., Kasten, E., Modini, S., Lettner, S., Baker, G., Persson, B. A., & Hessen, E. (2020). Clinical neuropsychology as a specialist profession in European health care: Developing a benchmark for training standards and competencies using the Europsy model? *Frontiers in Psychology, 11*. doi: 10.3389/fpsyg.2020.559134.

Karazsia, B. T., Stavnezer, A. J., & Reeves, J. W. (2013). Graduate admissions in Clinical Neuropsychology: The importance of undergraduate training. *Archives of Clinical Neuropsychology, 28*, 711–720.

Karazsia, B. T., & Smith, L (2016). Preparing for graduate-level training in professional psychology: Comparisons across PhD, Counseling PhD, and clinical PsyD programs. *Teaching of Psychology, 43*, 305–313. doi: 10.1177/0098628316662760

Kellogg, E. Cerbone, B, Kenealy, L., & Collins R. (2021). Preparing for and obtaining a predoctoral internship in neuropsychology. In C. K. Block (Ed.) *The neuropsychologist's roadmap: A training and career guide* (pages 33–54). American Psychological Association.

Kracen, A. C., & Wallace, I.J. (2008). *Applying to graduate school in psychology: Advice from successful students and prominent psychologists.* American Psychological Association.

National Institutes of Health (n.d.). *LRP Online Application.* U.S. Department of Health and Human Services. Retrieved January 29, 2023, from https://www.lrp.nih.gov/oas-welcome

Nelson, A. P., Roper, B. L., Slomine, B. S., Morrison, C., Greher, M. R., Janusz, J., Larson, J. C., Meadows, M-E., Ready, R. E., Rivera Mindt, M., Whiteside, D. M., Willment, K., & Wodushek, T. R. (2015). Official position of the American Academy of Clinical Neuropsychology (AACN): Guidelines for practicum training in clinical neuropsychology. *The Clinical Neuropsychologist, 29*(7), 879–904.

Norcross, J. C., & Sayette, M. A. (2022). *Insider's guide to graduate programs in clinical and counseling psychology* (2022/2023 edition). Guilford Press.

Perry, K. M., & Boccaccini, M. T. (2009). Specialized training in APA-accredited clinical psychology doctoral programs: Findings from a review of program websites. *Clinical Psychology: Science and Practice, 16*(3), 348.

Ponsford, J. (2017). International growth of neuropsychology. *Neuropsychology, 31*(8), 921.

Suhr, J., Woods, S. P., Alexander, C., & Babicz, M. (2021). Applying and getting into graduate school. In C. K. Block (Ed.) *The neuropsychologist's roadmap: A training and career guide* (pages 11–32). American Psychological Association.

Sweet, J. J., Klipfel, K. M., Nelson, N. W., & Moberg, P. J. (2021). Professional practices, beliefs, and incomes of U.S. neuropsychologists: The AACN, NAN, SCN 2020 practice and salary survey. *The Clinical Neuropsychologist, 35*, 7–80, doi: 10.1080/13854046.2020.1849803

Whiteside, D. M., Guidotti Breting, L. M., Butts, A. M., Hahn-Ketter, A. E., Osborn, K., Towns, S. J., Barisa, M., Santos, O.A., & Smith, D. (2016). 2015 American Academy of Clinical Neuropsychology (AACN) student affairs committee survey of neuropsychology trainees. *The Clinical Neuropsychologist, 30*, 664–694. doi: 10.1080/13854046.2016.1196731

6 Potential Difficulties and Challenges with a Career in Neuropsychology

Although hopefully it is obvious that we love the specialty of neuropsychology, like any career there are a few considerations or challenges of which you should be aware as you make your decision. Many of these are not unique to neuropsychology and may, in fact, be the same kinds of concerns you would encounter in one of the similar careers described in Chapter 2.

Training Is a Long Haul

As discussed in Chapter 5, a doctoral degree (either a Ph.D. or Psy.D.) is required to become a neuropsychologist. The fact that the doctorate is required *may* make the decision to complete that much schooling easier if you definitely want to go into the specialty, as opposed to neuroscience or another field where there is an option to stop at the Master's degree. Nevertheless, this is still a minimum 5–7-year commitment after college, followed by a postdoctoral fellowship of another two years, before you can start your "real" job. You do get paid on your internship and your fellowship, but these are typically in the $35–60K range respectively, well below what you will make as a professional psychologist. Don't underestimate the opportunity cost of not working while you're still in training those 7–9 years, any student loans you may have accrued, and the fact that many of your peers from undergraduate school will be out working while you are "still in school." Family and friends, too, may not truly understand what you're doing or why. In fact, most people do not know what a neuropsychologist is or does (you'll be describing what you do many times over), and many people cannot even correctly pronounce "*neuro*-psychologist." They may be on a different schedule than you (perhaps more of a 9–5 workday) and won't have to worry about writing papers, studying for exams, etc. You may find yourself envying those already working. The doctoral dissertation, especially, is something most people have never experienced, and it may be hard to find someone who understands or a sympathetic ear outside of your classmates. Research can take much, *much* longer than expected (especially if you change labs or projects), as can writing what will probably be the longest paper you have ever written in your life up to that point (it's a book, really).

DOI: 10.4324/9781003315513-6

Speaking of family, with such a long time in school typically overlapping with your mid to late 20s or early 30s, you may be wondering whether you will have to postpone having your own family, if that is something in which you are interested. This is a very personal decision. While having children during graduate school can certainly be done (one of your authors, LAS, did), you may have additional financial concerns (i.e., childcare) and it may prolong your training somewhat. Because externships/practica, internship, and fellowship are structured to have you work during a specific time period, this can be less than ideal timing to start a family, at least from your placement's point of view. Another consideration is, since family and school require competing demands on your time, you may find yourself being less able to spend time with your family and/or having to choose less rigorous training opportunities in order to do both.

Finally, the internship and postdoctoral fellowship, outlined in Chapter 5, may not end up being where you completed your doctoral training. Relocating, even temporarily, can be stressful, especially if you have a partner and/or children. If you love school, none of the above may be a problem, but – like medicine, or another career that takes many, many years of training – give serious thought to the above and make sure you have the resolve and determination (not to mention the financial resources) to commit to a doctorate and the subsequent training.

Continuing Education

Even once you have completed your doctorate, postdoctoral fellowship, license, and become board certified, you are still not "done." Licensing requires a certain number of Continuing Education (CE) credits every few years, depending on the state (as mentioned in Chapter 3). CE can be in the form of courses, seminars, workshops, journal readings, etc. Attendance at conferences can also count, and can be an enjoyable way to get CE credits while networking with peers. Board certification, too, requires maintenance of certification (MOC) every ten years, at least certification through the American Board of Professional Psychology (ABPP). MOC is not another exam; it is a process of self-examination and documentation of professional activities that demonstrate your continuing professional development. See the ABPP website listed in eResources for more information. Although CE and MOC do not require exams or grades, the learning for a neuropsychologist never ends.

Notes/Reports/Paperwork/Documentation

A common complaint of many neuropsychologists is the amount of time they spend writing reports. After each evaluation, the report may take another several hours, if they write it themselves (some neuropsychologists use dictation services or technicians). In addition, there is other paperwork, such as documentation of treatment sessions, notes that have to be entered into the electronic medical record, etc. This is certainly not something specific to neuropsychology, as many healthcare professions have experienced an increase in "paperwork" due to insurance issues, hospital compliance, government regulation, and legal liability. However, it can be exceedingly time consuming and may feel tedious, especially when (unlike a neuropsychological report) the notes are more cookie-cutter forms rather than something thought-provoking. Further, especially in private practice, time spent doing documentation is often not billable, meaning that these hours may come after, or on top of, hours you are already working. It should be noted that, in many settings, there is a trend toward shorter reports, for all of the reasons mentioned above as well as incentives by insurance companies to only pay for a fewer number of hours. Additionally, briefer, more targeted and efficient protocols can reduce wait-lists in areas with few neuropsychologists. Nevertheless, if you really hate to write for whatever reason, you may want to reconsider the specialty, given the lengthy dissertation you will write, followed by weekly (if not daily) reports.

Billing Issues /Insurance

Related to the documentation issue, billing requires time that is also typically not reimbursed. Negotiating with insurance companies for payment, coverage, or pre-authorization, can be extremely frustrating and time-consuming and not always fruitful. Ideally, whether in a hospital setting or private practice, someone else will be assigned this job. However, if you have a small private practice, you may be that person. Insurance companies can dictate the kinds of patients you see, for how long, and how much you are reimbursed, particularly if the patient's insurance is managed care. Reimbursement as a whole has been going down over the years. They can even refuse to include you on a provider panel. For this reason, some neuropsychologists in private practice refuse to accept some insurances and/or will try to balance the insurance patients they see with those who can pay out-of-pocket or with forensic cases, which can be more lucrative.

Time for Multiple Professional Activities

Chapter 3 discussed a variety of settings in which neuropsychologists can work. It also mentioned that many work in more than one role at a time. If one's primary work setting is a hospital or academic medical center, the neuropsychologist may also teach part-time and/or maintain a small private practice. This flexibility and variety were pointed out as strengths of the specialty. Nevertheless, these additional work roles may have to take place in the evenings and weekends, if the primary work setting is full-time. Finding time for "outside" writing, of journal articles, chapters, and books, is another challenge, if protected time for writing or research is not offered by the institution. Good time management and prioritization skills are essential. Of course, some neuropsychologists specialize and only do one thing. Concentrating on what one really wants to do will help prevent stress and feeling overwhelmed. However, saying "no" to additional opportunities takes some practice, and usually comes with experience, so that one does not suffer a fear of missing out.

Work-Life Balance

Speaking of stress, finding a healthy "balance" between work and personal life – family, friends, hobbies, etc. – is a challenge with any career (the word *balance* is really a misnomer). The good news is, compared to some related fields like medicine, neuropsychology does have controllable, fairly regular work hours. There are no real emergencies in neuropsychology, so you most likely would not have overnight "call" or have to work nights or weekends unless you wanted to. Nevertheless, working in a helping profession with sometimes difficult patients can be especially draining, and it is important to maintain good self-care and have support to prevent burnout. Self-care includes maintaining good sleep hygiene, eating well, keeping up with medical appointments, exercising, engaging in hobbies and pleasurable activities, and maintaining boundaries and prioritizing tasks. Support can include social interaction; it may also include individual psychotherapy or counseling for additional support. Regarding social interaction, other neuropsychologists can be great to network with, commiserate, and provide valuable input as to job-related concerns. However, having friends *outside* of neuropsychology can also provide a new perspective and may be a welcome reprieve if you want to discuss something besides work. See Feigon et al. (2018) for more discussion and ideas, for balance, and for finding time for multiple activities.

Work with Patients Can Be Difficult

As mentioned above, working with patients can be challenging and emotionally exhausting. Neuropsychologists work with patients suffering from neurological, medical, and/or psychiatric illness. As a result, they can exhibit behavioral symptoms which can be difficult to manage, such as childlike disinhibition (e.g., risky, inappropriate, or impulsive behavior), aggression, or refusal to participate in an evaluation or treatment. They can also be extremely anxious or depressed, crying throughout your interview or feeling suicidal. You may feel powerless to help them if, for example, they have suffered a very severe stroke and are unable to speak, or if you diagnose them with a dementia which will likely get worse. You may have to make tricky diagnostic decisions, or provide feedback to distraught patients or family members. In addition to behavioral and emotional symptoms, cognitive symptoms such as memory impairment can result in your patient not remembering their appointment or where to go. Or they may fail to follow through on recommendations. If a patient also has physical injuries (from, for example, an accident), you may have to tolerate looking at someone with a depressed skull fracture, someone who had brain surgery, was burned, or had an amputation. Patients may be unable to use part of their body, may be in a wheelchair, or be using a walker or cane. Determine in advance how you feel about working with people with disabilities, older adults, and/or sick children. You can utilize some of those self-care strategies discussed above, and discuss with your supervisor, colleagues, and/or your own therapist.

Limited Diversity

Neuropsychology, as in psychology as a whole, has lacked diversity. In recent years, there has been a shift from more males in the specialty to more females (Sweet et al., 2018), although males still make up the majority of leadership positions (Sachs et al., 2018). There are also a majority of non-Hispanic White practitioners and particularly amongst its leaders (Cory, 2021). This is especially problematic, given the diversity of the patients that we see and the implications for representative normative test data and the effect of healthcare disparities. However, neuropsychology has taken this seriously, and developed programs for improving equity, diversity, and inclusion (EDI) in psychology education and training (e.g., AACN's Relevance 2050 Initiative; SCN's Ethic and Minority Affairs Committee; Minnesota Conference). Websites for these are included in the eResources accompanying this book.

Scope of Practice Issues

A strength of neuropsychology is and has always been our *relationships* with patients, during interviews, evaluations, and therapy, and the empathy and sensitivity we demonstrate within that connection. Therefore, other professions taking on tasks of neuropsychologists (whether testing, therapy, cognitive remediation, or brain health education) and not performing them to our standards is problematic, and bad not only for the profession but for our patients. For example, some physician offices have taken to putting a patient alone in front of a computer for 20–30 minutes to take a "cognitive test," which is not at all thorough and not designed to be diagnostic, and then not providing them any feedback as to their performance. Although the goal there is to see more patients in a shorter amount of time, the practice lacks connection, education, and support for vulnerable patients. For other professions to attempt to replicate our services by trying to have computers do all the work takes out that relationship with patients and is simply bad care.

In some settings, like hospitals, other professions may also step on toes by performing a service outside their scope (i.e., testing or psychotherapy) which is better performed by neuropsychologists. Education offered to these professionals, as well as to patients, may help avert this. Another example is the corporate "brain health" industry, including over-the-counter pills/powders and computerized training that isn't rigorously validated to the standards of neuropsychology. This has resulted in numerous lawsuits for misleading advertising, ineffective if not dangerous products, and faulty information. Again, neuropsychologists are in the best position to provide education to patients and to the public about brain health, to help prevent any danger from these companies. We are the brain health experts; they are often simply trying to sell products.

In conclusion, like any profession, neuropsychology can have its challenges and potential issues. It is good to be aware of potential drawbacks before choosing a career, to determine whether some of the issues mentioned above apply to you or bother you personally. Alternatively, we hope we reassure you by saying that some issues may be minimized or prevented altogether with some preparation, and may be changing over time.

References

Cory, J. M. (2021). White privilege in neuropsychology: An 'invisible knapsack' in need of unpacking? *The Clinical Neuropsychologist, 35*(2), 206–218.

Feigon, M., Block, C., Guidotti Breting, L., Boxley, L., Dawson, E., & Cobia, D. (2018). Work–life integration in neuropsychology: A review of the existing literature and preliminary recommendations. *The Clinical Neuropsychologist, 32*(2), 300–317.

Sachs, B. C., Benitez, A., Buelow, M. T., Gooding, A., Schaefer, L. A., Sim, A. H., Tussey, C., & Shear, P. K. (2018). Women's leadership in neuropsychology: Historical perspectives, present trends, and future directions. *The Clinical Neuropsychologist, 32*(2), 217–234.

Sweet, J. J., Lee, C., Guidotti Breting, L. M., & Benson, L. M. (2018). Gender in clinical neuropsychology: Practice survey trends and comparisons outside the specialty. *The Clinical Neuropsychologist, 32*(2), 186–216.

7 Summary and Future Directions

While you begin the process of contemplating your career path and exploring options, we hope this book was helpful in introducing you to the exciting specialty of clinical neuropsychology, and in answering some of the questions you may have had. Here is a summary of the primary goals we had for this book:

Summary of Goals

1) *Defining the subject*: Neuropsychology is the study of brain and behavior, and combines the disciplines of biology (specifically neuroscience) and psychology (especially cognition). Clinical neuropsychology is a specialty within psychology, and specifically clinical psychology. Clinical neuropsychologists see patients across the lifespan for cognitive assessment, diagnosis, treatment, and/or rehabilitation.
2) *How to determine whether the career is a good fit*: When contemplating a career, you obviously want to do something in which you are interested and which plays to your strengths. A detailed self-analysis of your interests and strengths should include your skills and work values, but also your personality. Your school career office or academic advising may offer assessment of these and/or there are many tools available online. Other suggestions for career decision-making include reading up on the field, seeking out practical experiences, and speaking with others.
3) *Reviewing similar, complementary careers*: There are numerous related careers that are similar to or overlap with neuropsychology in some way. Reading about these and comparing them regarding their training and day-to-day activities should help you narrow down your choices.
4) *Describing what neuropsychologists do in different settings*: Neuropsychologists can work in many different settings including, but not limited to: hospital settings, rehabilitation centers, private practice, university teaching, research, industry, and forensic settings. Many neuropsychologists work in more than one of these settings. What neuropsychologists do will vary by setting, but there are some common activities.

DOI: 10.4324/9781003315513-7

5) *Reviewing the kinds of populations with whom neuropsychologists work*: The kinds of patients with whom clinical neuropsychologists work include patients with neurological, psychiatric, developmental, and/or medical illnesses and injuries across the lifespan.

6) *Outlining how one becomes a neuropsychologist*: It takes a long time to become a neuropsychologist, including time required to earn a doctoral degree in psychology. We review the training and describe how to become a neuropsychologist, including re-specialization from other careers. We also recommend a few first steps, if you are thinking about going down this path.

7) *Identifying potential challenges with this career*: As with any other career, there are some potential challenges with neuropsychology. Many are not unique to neuropsychology, and may be present in other healthcare fields and/or other professions which require extensive training. You should familiarize yourself with these when making your decision. However, we feel the pluses of being a neuropsychologist vastly outweigh the negatives.

Future Trends and Directions for Neuropsychology

Despite the potential challenges outlined in Chapter 6, we are optimistic of our specialty's ability to grow, evolve, and change with the times. Next, we will review some of the trends and areas of focus we anticipate seeing in the specialty of clinical neuropsychology in the near future.

Telepsychology

As discussed in Chapter 3, all neuropsychologists are trained to administer and interpret standardized tests of cognition that are developed using rigorous approaches. Until recently, the majority of our tests were developed for administration using paper-pencil formats. Computerized tests previously existed, and the transition to telehealth due to the COVID-19 pandemic is expected to accelerate research on the use of both new and existing tests in virtual formats. More training and treatment will likely be conducted virtually too. Telepsychology and its application to neuropsychology will therefore be an exciting new frontier to explore in the future.

Diversity

According to the U.S. Census Bureau (Vespa et al., 2020), it is projected that in the next 25 years there will no longer be a majority of White people in the United States. As many neuropsychological tests, especially the older ones, were standardized using people from White, English-speaking backgrounds, neuropsychologists are starting to address how our tests do and do not apply to people from other backgrounds, and how to improve our tools accordingly. This work is expected to continue into the future. In addition, as most neuropsychologists are currently White (Sweet et al., 2021) and predominantly English-speaking, greater effort will be put towards the cultivation of neuropsychology students from diverse backgrounds, and placing more of an emphasis in this area during graduate training. This process has already begun, for instance through the Relevance 2050 Initiative (American Academy of Clinical Psychology, 2022), discussed in Chapter 6. The recent Minnesota 2022 Update Conference (see https://minnesotaconference.org/), an update of the Houston Conference guidelines (mentioned in Chapter 5), has as its objective to seek to revise and extend education and training guidelines to increase diversity in training and in equitable access to neuropsychology research, education, and services. It also plans to integrate new developments in technology into neuropsychology. Finally, the training of neuropsychologists in mentorship and **sponsorship** (Hilsabeck, 2018), and particularly culturally-responsive mentorship (Calamia et al., 2022), is a goal for recruiting, retaining, and promoting trainees, especially of diverse backgrounds. A current example, the New2Neuropsychology initiative (https://new2neuropsych.org), has as its mission outreach to historically underrepresented students, and can connect students with a mentor or student liaison. If you already speak another language or languages besides English, this can be a real strength, and you should take advantage of this and emphasize this skill when applying to programs.

Advances in Medicine

The field of medicine is ever-changing and advancing, both in the development of innovative treatments and cures, but also in the appearance of new diseases and syndromes. In the area of cancer, for instance, the cognitive implications of **"chemo brain"** have become well-recognized. There has also been rapid expansion in the use of new treatments such as immunotherapies and stem cell therapies which have dramatically increased survival rates for some cancers with previously poor prognoses, but less is known about the physical, cognitive, and emotional impacts of these treatments or long-term survivorship of these illness. Our skills as neuropsychologists would apply perfectly to investigating possible implications on the brain and then addressing them.

In addition, the COVID-19 pandemic highlights the potential for new diseases to emerge which can impact the brain either directly or indirectly. From the beginning of the pandemic, neuropsychologists quickly utilized our skills to better understand and address the impact of COVID-19 and "long COVID" in terms of cognitive and emotional functioning. Similar work can be conducted with any illness in the future with the potential to impact the brain.

Focus on Prevention and Brain Health

Despite advances, we know that some diseases and conditions, such as dementia, currently cannot be reversed once clinically significant. Thus, one trend in neuropsychology is a shift toward the promotion of brain health and the *prevention* of cognitive decline, rather than focusing solely on diagnosis and treatment/management. As mentioned in Chapter 6, neuropsychologists are brain health experts. We utilize scientific research to educate others, patients and public alike, about activities proven to enhance cognitive functioning and prevent or stave off decline. These "brain health" activities include exercise, maintaining a healthy diet and weight, managing health issues like hypertension or diabetes, reducing or eliminating effects of smoking and alcohol, stress management, attaining quality sleep, socialization, and cognitive activity. While not new ideas, many people falsely consider the brain ("mind") and the body to be separate, and are surprised to find out that what is good for the body is also good for the brain, and vice versa. Some are disappointed, wanting to rely on some newly touted pill or game or product to improve their memory or prevent dementia. This public health role for neuropsychologists will become increasingly important as the population ages (and the environment becomes more toxic), and is an area where we can contribute a lot given our knowledge and skills.

Title Protection for Neuropsychology

In the U.S., all states have a licensing procedure to be able to practice psychology independently and use the title "psychologist." Of note, in some states, those with a doctorate in psychology who solely perform academic work such as teach at a university and/or work in a research facility (i.e., do not see patients clinically) may be exempt from having to attain a license. Licensing, however, is generic and does not denote competence in a specialty; most states do not have a license specific for neuropsychologists, or any other specialty. Currently, board certification is the only way to indicate to peers and the public that one has attained competence in clinical neuropsychology (Cox and Grus, 2019). Advocacy is underway on a state-by-state basis to try to obtain title protection for neuropsychology by having specialty licenses. The hope is to prevent people without specialized training from misleading the public by referring to themselves as neuropsychologists. Specialty licensing could also be of benefit when dealing with insurance companies.

Final Thoughts

Our aim for this book was to serve as a resource guide for your career exploration and decision-making. We remember – it can be nerve-wracking to narrow down and choose a career, and there is a lot invested. We love and are enthusiastic about psychology, and working with and thinking about the brain, and you must too if you picked up this book! Neuropsychologists have both curious and caring personalities. While we hope we've inspired you to consider the fascinating and rewarding path of neuropsychology, we thank you for learning more about our specialty and wish you luck on your journey!

References

American Academy of Clinical Neuropsychology (2022). *Relevance 2050 Initiative.* https://theaacn.org/relevance-2050/relevance-2050-initiative/

Calamia, M., Kaseda, E. T., Price, J. S., De Vito, A., Silver, C. H., Cherry, J., VanLandingham, H., Khan, H., Sparks, P.J., & Ellison, R. L. (2022). Mentorship in clinical neuropsychology: Survey of current practices, cultural responsiveness, and untapped potential. *Journal of Clinical and Experimental Neuropsychology, 44*(5–6), 366–385.

Cox, D. R., & Grus, C. L. (2019). From continuing education to continuing competence. *Professional Psychology: Research and Practice, 50*(2), 113.

Hilsabeck, R. C. (2018). Comparing mentorship and sponsorship in clinical neuropsychology. *The Clinical Neuropsychologist, 32*(2), 284–299.

Sweet, J. J., Klipfel, K. M., Nelson, N. W., & Moberg, P. J. (2021). Professional practices, beliefs, and incomes of U.S. neuropsychologists: The AACN, NAN, SCN 2020 practice and "salary survey." *The Clinical Neuropsychologist, 35,* 7–80, doi: 10.1080/13854046.2020.1849803

Vespa, J., Medina, L., & and Armstrong, D. M. (2020). Demographic Turning Points for the United States: Population Projections for 2020 to 2060. *Current Population Reports*, P25–1144, U.S. Census Bureau, Washington, D.C.

Glossary

Abulia   Lack of initiation or motivation, due to changes in the brain.

Academic   Related to school.

Accredited   An approval process by the American Psychological Association. Doctoral programs (and internships) must meet certain standards to earn this approval.

Behavioral neurologist   Similar to neuropsychiatrists, but come to the field from neurology (after an additional fellowship after residency), rather than psychiatry. Focus more on cognitive impairment and aphasia in patients with injuries and illnesses to the brain.

Behavioral neuroscience   Branch of neuroscience examining the relationship between the nervous system and behavior, cognition, and emotion.

"Chemo brain"   Cognitive difficulties and brain-related fatigue that some people experience following chemotherapy.

Clinical health psychologist (or health psychologist)   Doctoral-level psychologist that examines how biological, social, and psychological factors influence health and illness, and seeks to prevent illness and promote health. Clinical health psychologists work clinically, whereas health psychologists may be more involved in research.

Clinical neuropsychologist   Doctoral-level psychologist that has expertise in brain-behavior relationships and uses this knowledge in the assessment, diagnosis, treatment, and/or rehabilitation of those with neurological, medical, developmental, psychiatric, and learning disorders. Clinical neuropsychologists typically have a degree in clinical psychology (occasionally counseling psychology) with additional specialized training in neuropsychology.

Clinical psychologist   Doctoral-level psychologist that assesses, diagnoses, and treats mental, emotional, and behavioral issues, and works with patients with anxiety, depression, psychosis, personality disorders, eating disorders, addictions, learning disabilities, and family or relationship issues.

Cognition   Thinking skills, including processing speed, attention, memory, language, visuospatial functioning, organization, planning, and problem-solving that neuropsychologists typically test using standardized tests.

Cognitive remediation   A form of treatment where patients are trained in strategies that can help improve cognitive skills like attention, memory, and organization.

Continuing Education (CE)   Participation in educational events so that psychologists can keep their licenses to practice.

Counseling psychologist   Doctoral-level psychologist that works with less severe types of psychopathologies, may provide vocational counseling, and tends to be employed in university or community counseling centers.

Dissertation   An original research project that is required to earn a doctoral degree. The standards depend largely on the individual program and mentor. Sometimes referred to as a "thesis," although thesis is typically reserved for the research project to earn a Master's degree.

Early intervention   Services like speech or physical therapy that can be offered to babies or pre-school-aged children for various delays or disabilities.

Eclectic   Integrating a variety of schools of thought. An "eclectically" oriented doctoral program may incorporate training in both Cognitive Behavioral Therapy and psychodynamic psychotherapy.

Externship (also called a **practicum**)   A part-time clinical training experience, usually at a hospital, clinic, or school. Doctoral students usually complete at least two of these during their training, and they are typically unpaid.

Forensic neuropsychologist   Clinical neuropsychologist who has had training and experience to work within forensic settings (i.e., courts, prisons/jails, with attorneys, etc.).

Forensic psychologist   Doctoral-level psychologist that examines individuals who are involved with the legal system and may work within prisons or in court settings.

Geropsychologist   Doctoral-level psychologist who specializes in the care of older adults.

Grand Rounds   Lectures, often given at academic medical centers, by professors, researchers, or clinicians who work in specialized medical areas.

Health psychologist   See *clinical health psychologist.*

Impulsivity   Acting without thinking.

Internship   A one-year paid training position that a doctoral student must complete towards the end of his/her training.

Learning   Taking in and keeping new information to use later on. Requires several cognitive skills, including attention, understanding of information, and memory.

Marriage and family therapist   Mental health clinician who assesses, diagnoses, and treats psychological distress within the context of the marriage, couple, and family systems.

Mental health counselor   Mental health clinician who sees patients with anxiety, depression, substance issues, and relationship issues. They are less likely than clinical psychologists to see patients with severe psychopathology.

Mentorship Guidance and support provided to a student or trainee by someone with more experience, for the purposes of personal and/or professional growth.

Neurodiagnostic technologist (also, surgical neurophysiologist) Healthcare professionals that work under the oversight of a physician (neurologist or surgeon), typically in a hospital and not infrequently in an operating room. They are responsible for intraoperative neuromonitoring during surgery on the brain, spine, or nerves, and may also perform EEGs, EMGs and other tests.

Neurologist Physician who focuses on the brain and nervous system; examines more basic functions like sensation, reflexes, and muscle strength, with higher cognitive functions typically limited to a brief mental status examination.

Neuropsychiatrist Neuropsychiatrists are psychiatrists with additional fellowship training. Evaluate and treat injuries and diseases of the brain, focusing on psychiatric, behavioral, and emotional disorders (such as psychosis, impulsivity, abulia, etc.) arising from neurological injury or illness.

Neuropsychology A specialty of psychology examining the relationship between brain structure and function and behavior.

Neuroscience The study of the nervous system, including the brain.

Occupational therapist Helps people with disabilities, both by restoring and improving their ability to accomplish daily activities at home and at work and by assisting with accommodations to support accessibility.

Pediatric Related to children or adolescents, especially in the medical field.

Pediatric neuropsychologist Clinical neuropsychologist who has had training and experience to work especially or solely with children and adolescents (sub-specialty of neuropsychology).

Physiatrist Physician who coordinates physical medicine and rehabilitation.

Postdoctoral fellowship Sometimes referred to as a "residency," the formal training program that takes place after earning the doctoral degree (for board certification in clinical neuropsychology, the equivalent of a two-year fellowship is required).

Practicum See *externship.*

Problem-solving Using skills to figure out how to best manage new situations.

Progressive condition A condition that gets worse over time.

Psychiatrist Physician that focuses on mood, psychotic, addictive, behavior, and personality disorders, and treats patients with mental illnesses such a schizophrenia, major depressive disorder, bipolar disorder, and obsessive-compulsive disorder.

Psychology The scientific study of the mind, mental processes, and behavior.

Psychometrician   A job where somebody administers neuropsychological tests to people in a clinical or research setting. This is done under the supervision of a licensed neuropsychologist.

Rehabilitation psychologist   Doctoral-level psychologist with specialized training to work with patients with disabilities and chronic health conditions.

Reliability   Degree to which test results or scores are consistent from one administration to another; their stability and precision.

Re-specialize   To change your specialty area, especially after having already received training or specialized in another (usually related) area.

Risk factor   Anything in the person's medical history, family history, or other things about a person like age, ethnicity, or sex that put a person at higher risk for a certain medical condition.

School psychologist   Psychologist that works within the educational system (often elementary, middle, and high schools) to help children and adolescents with emotional, social, and learning issues. Required training and practice varies somewhat by state.

Sensorimotor skills   Skills that require the five senses (sight, hearing, touch, taste, and smell) to perceive or understand the world.

Social worker   Clinician who can be employed in a variety of settings, including hospitals, social service agencies, schools, and private practice. They work with people with mental illnesses and emotional disturbances, marital and family difficulties, substance abuse, behavioral and learning disorders of children and adolescents, and community problems and social issues.

Speech and Language Pathologist   Clinician who diagnoses, evaluates, and treats disorders of speech, voice, swallowing, and/or language.

Sponsorship   Making connections and advocating for a trainee for the purposes of advancing their career; sponsors typically have some clout or are in positions of influence.

Standardized tests   Tests that are created by being given in the same way to large groups of "practice" people to determine what would be an average score, an above average score, or a below average score when given to real clients.

Stipend   A small salary that a doctoral student may earn for working in a research lab or teaching.

Surgical neurophysiologist   See *neurodiagnostic technologist.*

Validity   Degree to which a test measures what it is supposed to measure; its accuracy.

Wada procedure   When a medication (intracarotid sodium amobarbital) is injected to temporarily "put the brain to sleep" one hemisphere at a time, to determine in which side of the brain language and memory abilities are located.

Index

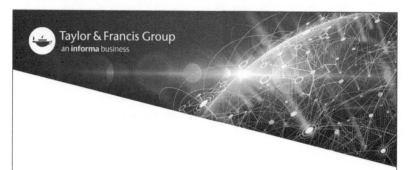